Eat Fat

MW00475559

The Beginners Guide To Successfully Transitioning To An Eat Fat Get Thin, Ketogenic Diet For Rapid Weight Loss

With 100+ Simple And Delicious Recipes

© Copyright 2016 by David Wilson - All rights reserved.

This document is geared towards providing exact and reliable information in regards to the topic and issue covered. The publication is sold with the idea that the publisher is not required to render accounting, officially permitted, or otherwise, qualified services. If advice is necessary, legal or professional, a practiced individual in the profession should be ordered.

- From a Declaration of Principles which was accepted and approved equally by a Committee of the American Bar Association and a Committee of Publishers and Associations.

In no way is it legal to reproduce, duplicate, or transmit any part of this document in either electronic means or in printed format. Recording of this publication is strictly prohibited and any storage of this document is not allowed unless with written permission from the publisher. All rights reserved.

The information provided herein is stated to be truthful and consistent, in that any liability, in terms of inattention or otherwise, by any usage or abuse of any policies, processes, or directions contained within is the solitary and utter responsibility of the recipient reader. Under no circumstances will any legal responsibility or blame be held against the publisher for any reparation, damages, or monetary loss due to the information herein, either directly or indirectly.

Respective authors own all copyrights not held by the publisher.

The information herein is offered for informational purposes solely, and is universal as so. The presentation of the information is without contract or any type of guarantee assurance.

The trademarks that are used are without any consent, and the publication of the trademark is without permission or backing by the trademark owner. All trademarks and brands within this book are for clarifying purposes only and are the owned by the owners themselves, not affiliated with this document.

Medical Disclaimer

You understand that any information as found within this book is for general educational and informational purposes only. You understand that such information is not intended nor otherwise implied to be medical advice.

You understand that such information is by no means complete or exhaustive, and that as a result, such information does not encompass all conditions, disorders, health-related issues, or respective treatments. You understand that you should always consult your physician or other healthcare provider to determine the appropriateness of this information for your own situation or should you have any questions regarding a medical condition or treatment plan.

This information has not been evaluated or approved by the FDA and is not necessarily based on scientific evidence from any source. These statements have not been evaluated by the Food and Drug Administration (FDA). The products referred to in the book are intended to support general well-being and are not intended to treat, diagnose, mitigate, prevent, or cure any condition or disease.

You agree not to use any information in our book, including, but not limited to product descriptions, customer testimonials, etc. for the diagnosis and treatment of any health issue or for the prescription of any medication or treatment.

You acknowledge that all customer testimonials as found on in our book are strictly the opinion of that person and any results such person may have achieved are solely individual in nature; your results may vary.

You understand that such information is based upon personal experience and is not a substitute for obtaining professional medical advice. You should always consult your physician or other healthcare provider before changing your diet or starting an exercise program.

In light of the foregoing, you understand and agree that we are not liable nor do we assume any liability for any information contained within our book as well as your reliance on it. In no event shall we be liable for direct, indirect, consequential, special, exemplary, or other damages related to your use of the information contained within our book.

Copyright © Orion Systems

David Wilson's Publications

Below you'll find some of my other books that are popular on Amazon and Kindle as well. Simply go to the links below to find out more. Alternatively, you can visit my author page on Amazon to see other work done by me.

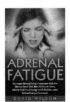 Adrenal Fatigue: Overcome Adrenal Fatigue Syndrome With The Adrenal Reset Diet. How To Reduce Stress, Anxiety And Boost Energy Levels And Overcome Adrenal Fatigue Syndrome

Go to: http://amzn.to/1U1a1GH

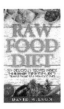 Raw Food Diet: 50+ Raw Food Recipes Inside This Raw Food Cookbook. Raw Food Diet For Beginners In This Step By Step Guide To Successfully Transitioning To A Raw Food Diet

Go to: http://amzn.to/1OgfXyJ

If the links do not work, for whatever reason, you can simply search for these titles on the Amazon website to find them.

Table of Contents

Buttered Rasher-Wrapped Sausages

Spicy Steak Bites

Baked Beef Curry

Brussels Sprout Chips

Curried Cabbage and Broccoli

Cabbage and Mushroom Stroganoff

Low Carb Crock Pot Chili

Parmesan Cauliflower Soup

Teriyaki Fried Brown Lentils with Chicken

Cauliflower Tabbouler

Creamy Chicken and Peppers Enchilada

Slow Cooker Thai Beef with Roasted Cauliflower (serves 4)

Sun-Dried Tomato Turkey and Dried Tomato Burgers with Avocado

Chicken Dijonnaise

Baked Garlic and Cheese Chicken

Oven Baked Rabbit Dijon

Spiced Salmon with Chili Sauce

Cabbage Roll Stew

Lamb and Mushrooms

Beef and Veggie Stuffed Peppers

Venison and Mushrooms

Fish and Baby Tomato Bake

Sautéed Minute Steaks

Broiled Tilapia Parmesan

Sweet Potato Fritters

Roasted Portobello Mushrooms

Butternut Cups

Cheesy Beef Cauliflower

Slow Cooked Tilapia Cheese

Chili Chicken with Mushroom

Sweet Potato Fish Cakes

Cauliflower Tabbouleh Salad

Buttered Garlic Cauliflower Mash

Steak with Fried Tomatoes

Spiced Chicken Curry

Veal and Shallot Casserole with Sage and Mushrooms

Tandoori Chicken

Peppered Beef Chickoli

Slow Cooked Low Carb Mexi Chicken

Slow Cooker Lamb Carnitas

Zucchini Cake with Whipped Cream

Pumpkin Cake with Whipped Cream

Baby Spinach and Eggs

Savory Lentil Cake

Veal and Mushrooms

Crisp Roast Butternut

Slow Cooked Fish Cakes

Jicama Noodle Salad and Creamy Tahini-Ginger

Thai Chili Prawns with Courgette Noodles

Grilled Salmon and Boiled Sweet Potato

Baked Sweet Potatoes

Pesto Chicken and Brown Mushrooms on Zucchini Noodles

Rabbit Meat Panfry

BBQ Chickpeas and Cilantro Humus with Asparagus, Avocado and Sweet Potato

Guacamole Burgers on Portobello Mushrooms

Veal Chops with Mushrooms and Couscous

Five Spice Salmon Fillets with Sesame Cabbage

Butternut and Coconut Cake (serves 6)

Sealed Hake with Olive Salsa

Spaghetti Squash and Chickpea Sauce

Shawarma Chicken with Basil-Lemon Vinaigrette

Beef and Broccoli Stir-fry

Caesar Salad

Paleo Scotch Eggs

Onion Rings

Spicy Gizzards

Homemade Black Berry Chocolate

Guilt-free Brussels Sprout Chips

Multi-berry Roll-Ups

Macadamia Nut Hummus

Turkey Bacon-Wrapped Eggplant

Fried Chili Onion Rings

Sweet Potato Roast

Nutty Butter and Berry Bites

Parsnip Chips with Truffle Oil

Chocolate Cherry Bites

Fried Eggplant

Roasted Pumpkin Seeds

Roasted Cauliflower

Vanilla and Almond Chia Pudding

Introduction

I want to thank you and congratulate you for purchasing the book, *"Eat Fat Get Thin: The Beginners Guide To Successfully Transitioning To An Eat Fat Get Thin, Ketogenic Diet For Rapid Weight Loss With 100+ Simple And Delicious Recipes"*.

This book contains proven steps and strategies on how to get thin while eating fat, contrary to the popular and age old belief that fat makes you obese. The book provides easy to follow recipes that are guaranteed to see you rapidly lose unwanted excess pounds if you strictly follow the said diet. The following are some of the direct benefits obtainable from the information in this book:

- Exciting, delicious, nutritious and health packed recipes for the special occasions, for home alone meals and even for those times when you can't think of what to cook and are at the danger of resorting to the unhealthy take away meals.
- Explanations on the concept behind the "Eat fat Get Healthy" allure.
- You are taken on a journey through the first few weeks of taking this bull by the horns and guided through the issues you may face.
- A detailed explanation about how the diet works, including, but not limited to the physiological and biochemical changes occurring in the body as a result of the diet.

This list is not comprehensive but is merely a peek at what the book offers. More information awaits you as you start reading.

Thanks again for purchasing this book, I hope you enjoy it!

Eat Fat Get Thin; What Is It?

This is the name of the program developed by Dr. Mark Hyman after many years of research into the health benefits of fats and the many myths behind the world's minimal consumption of fat. According to Dr. Hyman, Science misled the world into demonizing fats for so long, leaving the real culprits behind our health complications and problems, sugar and starch, enjoying their undisturbed havoc upon us.

This program from Dr. Hyman is meant to correct the wrongs and the misconceptions about fat and tell the world that sugar and starch, and not fat, are the real reasons behind world obesity and disease. It is meant to guide people into eating good fats and ditching empty carbs for that desired change in their health. It provides guidelines into the right and healthy fats to eat to ensure you get the body you desire and shed those unwanted pounds obtained from eating lots of empty carbohydrates, non-food items and too much sugar.

As you follow Dr. Hyman's plan, you will be eating the delicious things you have been told are not good for you, and this time, you know "fat from fiction" to quote the doctor; and you can begin to achieve the body you desire.

Dr. Hyman's diet plan is based on the different processes our bodies go through depending on the type of food you are consuming. When you consume a diet rich in fats as opposed to carbs, your body burns body fat to use for energy because there is no other source of fuel that would otherwise be readily available if you were to consume lots of carbs. As a result of these processes, it makes sense to EFGT.

The old common misconception that more fat will make you obese yet carbohydrates are in fact the culprit has now been dealt with effectively through the provision of information from the main proponent of the EFGT diet. Not only is there enough scientific evidence to back the research up, many people are already living the life of eating fat to get thin and they are doing just that, eating fat and getting thin! There are some things that you just can't deny and this is one of those. It matters not that we have been made to believe the contrary for so many years, the truth is now among us and we should live by it. Go on and enjoy the good fats in your diet and give up the real troublemakers: carbohydrates in both sugar and starch form.

How the EFGT diet works

Our bodies' main source of energy is carbohydrates. When we eat food with too much carbohydrate we give the body enough to convert to glucose for its use in a process called glycolysis and even provide additional energy that is stored as fat for use when there is a drought of carbohydrates to convert to glucose. This is the reason why a diet high in carbs will lead to weight gain.

If you haven't eaten, e.g. you just woke up, your body still needs energy to use and therefore there is a reversal of glycolysis, a process called gluconeogenesis where the body converts non-carbohydrate sources like amino acids in the liver into energy for emergency purposes - this does not promote body fat burning.

However, when you eat a diet high in fat and very low in carbs like the EFGT diet, your body has no carbohydrates to convert to glucose and therefore the body is forced to burn the reserved energy stores, i.e. your body fat, in a process called ketosis. When ketosis occurs, your body will be using the excess fat, so you lose fat and consequently, the weight that goes with it. So you see, it makes sense to chuck out those carbs and stick to fat to burn fat.

A guide on how to start the EFGT diet, in brief: A rough 21-day plan

It is recommended that in the two days prior to starting the program, you should set aside a day each for getting rid of the bad stuff in your house to ensure that no temptations will overcome you. Such things like sugar and its products, flour and its products, alcohol, processed and factory made foods, liquid sugar calories in drinks, and even most types of beans. If you remove the temptations and are required to seek out those tempting foods elsewhere, it will be easier and require less willpower than if you just had to open the fridge.

The next thing you'll want to do is collect and prepare the proper things in order to get started. Go out and shop for what you will need for the first few days to ensure you do not get frustrated very early in the game, as this may lead to demotivation and frustration.

What is expected of you within that period?

This plan is based on a particular diet, so nutrition and your choices of food will play a pivotal role. You are, therefore, expected to eat the recommended foods and the quantities thereof. You can eat meat, with its fat on – tastes much better than lean, anyway. You can eat your good fats from the nuts, avocados, etc. You can eat an unlimited quantity of vegetables like kale, cabbage, broccoli, cauliflower, asparagus, artichokes, collard greens, dandelion greens, eggplant, endive, and many others with low starch content. You should always have vegetables making up ½ to ¾ of your plate, then the remaining part as a protein and very little carbohydrates. Eat your eggs, as long as they are organic. Meat should be from grass-fed beef, etc.

Health is not only about the food you eat, but also your activity level. **Exercise,** therefore, takes up a large part of a healthy life. We are not talking serious exercising, like lifting weights, but easy to do exercises like 30-minute walks, etc. You will be surprised just how much of an improvement you'll experience from a thirty-minute walk every day. The plan expects you to do some minimal exercises to go with the diet, so go for it!

You cannot rely just on your eyes and feelings to tell you whether or not something is materializing from the plan. Both eyes and feelings can lie and so you'll need to **keep a diary of everything that takes place** in relation to the 21-day plan. You are expected to write your beginning weight, height, waist size and such and then you should measure these during the course of the plan and record them. This is the most reliable way of knowing what is going on with your body. Not only do you record your weight, but even track your feelings, your thoughts and your experiences as a way to track how a healthy lifestyle will improve various facets of your life. Write about that. You never know where your motivation will come from.

For you to effectively undertake the EFGT plan to the end, you'll need to be sure you get enough sleep. Sleep is one aspect of life most people neglect, but not so when you are undergoing this plan. Sleep is essential for health and as such, you should give sleep its due time. It is during sleep that your damaged body tissues are repaired and your mind processes things that took place while you were awake. To help your body achieve its optimum state of health, try to sleep for 7 to 9 hours a night.

The supplements recommended for you to take with the program can also be quite helpful, so don't forget the importance of the supplements.

Suggestions of your daily schedule from Dr. Mark Hyman's EFGT manual:

YOUR 21-DAY SCHEDULE

Morning:

Begin the day with 30 minutes of brisk walking
Before breakfast, take 2 to 5 grams of the PGX fiber: 1 to 2 packets or ½ to 1 scoop of the powder in 10 ounces of water
Take your supplements with breakfast
Make your shake or breakfast
Enjoy a mid-morning snack (optional)
Drink water (at least 8 glasses throughout the day)

Afternoon:

Before lunch, take 2.5 to 5 grams of the PGX fiber
Eat lunch
Enjoy a mid-afternoon snack (optional)
Drink water (at least 8 glasses throughout the day)

Evening:

Spend 15 minutes recording your experience in your journal. Write down how you feel, any improvements or changes in your energy and focus, and how these changes make you feel physically, mentally, and emotionally

Practice deep breathing exercises for 5 minutes (or do this before each meal). Potato starch (optional) 1 TBSP in water before bed. It is a resistant starch that helps grow healthy bacteria in the gut and also enhances stage 4 deep sleep.

Get 7-8 hours of sleep

CHECKLIST FOR PHASE TWO:

- Follow the menus and recipes for breakfast, lunch and dinner (or use the simple cooking suggestions as an alternative).
- Take your supplements as directed (PGX before every meal and the rest with breakfast – take just before you eat).
- Plan your 30 minutes of exercise – brisk walking is fine and the more better. Record your experience and thoughts daily in your journal.
- Schedule your relaxation time - remember it's only 5 minutes!

Experiences, symptoms and obstacles found along the road to health with EFGT

You obviously know that as you work with this plan, a lot of changes will take place in your body. Among them will be pleasurable feelings as you start to experience a no FLC life, but with the good will also come the bad. There are some common and unpleasant symptoms that you may, or may not have. There are experiences that many face and for some, there are obstacles, which may be encountered and if not prepared for, your plans could be jeopardized.

The number one obstacle most people have to face is **getting rid of the old thinking that fat is bad and replacing it with new thinking**. Many times, those following the plan find themselves trimming off the fat from the meat because this is what they have always done and now its second nature. Before the new belief can to take root, the old has to be removed to make room for the new.

Dr. Hyman suggests that a day before you start the EFGT plan, you should throw away all the stuff in your cupboards that is not aligned with the plan. As easy as this may seem, it can still be a rough ride, at least in the first few days. A complete and sudden withdrawal from most things one is used to eating can lead to withdrawal symptoms like stomach pain, headache, nausea, irritation and frustration, etc.

Some people follow the plan blindly without **getting necessary guidance or enough information from Dr. Hyman**'s team or writings. Lack of information has the potential to ruin even the best of intentions. The EFGT plan has some basic rules that one should follow to make the journey easier, and without this info, someone might find that there is no progress being made. There is a great deal of information about the plan, but the key lies in knowing where to find it. Brush up on Dr. Hyman's books, blogs and articles to receive more in-depth, and continued guidance.

The **desire to lose all excess weight in a week** because you are following a diet guaranteed to work is not helpful because it is setting the bar unreasonably and impossibly high. Losing weight is good. In fact, it is the reason why the majority of people are using this plan. But you must give it enough time to happen in due course. Avoid limiting yourself too much or driving your body too hard as this might reverse the gains of the plan. Expect to lose weight some days and have no weight change or even slight gains on some days; it's all in the game. Relax and enjoy the food. Weight loss will come. Be patient.

Some may feel nothing is happening even though they are sticking to the plan. Even if everyone around you is losing weight, there is no guarantee that you will lose at the same time or with the same rate. Our physiological make-up is different from that of the next person, so we all weight loss (or gain) at a different rate. Don't let this discourage you! Just keep fighting the good fight and you will surely achieve that which you are striving for, whether it is better health and/or weight loss.

Supplements to use with EFGT plan

Our bodies require fiber, photo-nutrients, minerals, and vitamins to allow us to   function at our maximum. Supplements and nutrients help speed up weight loss by curbing our runaway appetites and by providing vital components to assist in gearing our metabolic systems to function properly and efficiently. It is, therefore, so unfortunate that most of our diets these days lack these essential components and lead to deficiencies that drive us into crazy cravings and frequent hunger pangs. But, thanks should be given to science for providing supplements to deal with these deficiencies.

As you get into the *21 day Eat Fat, Get Thin* plan, you may need these supplements more than most because of the chemical reactions your body will be undergoing as a result of dietary changes. Dr. Hyman foresaw this and prepared simple and easy to take supplements to ease your transition and progress. Among the supplements he recommends during the plan are:

- Magnesium citrate, which helps prevent constipation, muscle cramps, assists in sleep and is generally believed to be necessary in controlling blood sugar levels. Maintaining stable blood sugars is especially necessary as you change diets.
- EPA/DHA is an omega 3 fatty acid that is both pure and free of toxins, which the good doctor also recommends as part of the plan.
- Vitamin D3 is also one of the recommended supplements and similar to EPA/ DHA. This vitamin helps reverse what Dr. Hyman calls diabesity.
- Dr. Hyman's last recommendation is a super fiber believed to curb appetite, reduce blood sugar swings and help in weight loss. This supplement, known as PGX, must be mixed with cold water and taken before main meals.

The suggested supplement dosages are:

- Multivitamin - 2 a day
- Vitamin D3 - 2000 to 4000 IU a day

- Omega 3 fats (EPA/DHA) - 2 grams a day
- PGX - 2.5 to 5 grams before every meal in a large glass of water
- Magnesium citrate - 300 mg at night. Magnesium glycinate is recommended if you develop or are inclined to loose stool.
- MCT Oil or organic coconut oil - 1-2 tablespoon daily minimum
- Potato starch - 1 tablespoon in cold water at bedtime

You can use the following recipes after the first 14 days of your EFGT plan

Breakfast Recipes

Frittata (serves 4)

Ingredients

- 6 ounces spinach, chopped
- 7 ounces chopped Portobello mushrooms
- 1 tablespoon macadamia oil
- 3 chopped asparagus spears
- 1/2 cup diced white onion
- 6 large organic eggs
- 1 teaspoon black pepper
- 1 teaspoon sea salt

Method

1) Preheat oven to 180°C.
2) In an oven-safe skillet, heat 1/2 tablespoon coconut oil over medium heat.
3) Stir-fry vegetables for 3 minutes, until onion looks clear and the mushrooms are soft.
4) Remove vegetables from heat and set aside.
5) Whisk eggs in a large mixing bowl and stir in the vegetables.
6) Heat 1/2 tablespoon macadamia oil in the oven-safe skillet over medium-low heat.
7) Pour frittata mixture into the skillet and slow cook for 4–5 minutes.
8) Place frittata in the oven and bake for 10 minutes, or until frittata feels spongy but still firm to the touch.
9) Cut to desired size and serve.

Turkey and Macadamia Frittata (serves 4)

Ingredients

- 3 teaspoons macadamia oil
- 1/2 cup red peppers, chopped
- 1/3 cup chopped onion
- 3 slices crispy Turkey bacon, chopped
- 2 cups de-stemmed, rinsed and chopped kale
- 8 large organic eggs
- 1/2 cup coconut milk
- Sea salt and pepper for seasoning

Method

1) Preheat oven to 175° C.
2) Whisk eggs and coconut milk together in a medium sized bowl.
3) Add sea salt and pepper and set aside.
4) Heat half the macadamia oil in a thick based skillet (oven friendly) over medium heat and add onions and red pepper.
5) Stir-fry for 3 minutes or so, or until onion is clear.
6) Stir in kale and fry for five minutes, it should be wilted by then.
7) Add eggs and Turkey bacon to the mixture in the skillet.
8) Allow to cook for about 4 minutes; the bottom and edges of the frittata will start to set.
9) Put skillet in the oven and bake frittata for 10-15 minutes until it is thoroughly cooked.
10) Cut into slices or as desired and serve.

Turkey Bacon, Egg and No-Bread Sandwich
(serves 2)

Ingredients

- 2 tablespoons macadamia oil
- 2 cups sliced red bell peppers and cauliflower
- 3 large organic eggs
- 4 slices Turkey bacon

Method

1) Heat the macadamia oil in a thick based frying pan at medium heat.
2) Add the veggies and stir-fry until softened and until all liquid evaporates.
3) Remove from heat and use same pan to fry the bacon.
4) In the meantime, heat oil in another pan and fry the bacon.
5) Reduce the heat to low on the vegetable pan then remove from heat.
6) Flatten the vegetables and move them to the center of the pan.
7) Beat and add eggs to the vegetable pan, ensure the eggs are evenly spread around the pan and that the egg mixture touches the sides of the pan.
8) Put the eggs and veggies' pan back to the stove.
9) Check to see if bacon is cooked, remove from the pan and drain off excess fat.
10) Neatly slice each piece half-ways and set aside.
11) Turn to the egg mixture, which should no longer be bubbling. When the edges have pulled away from the sides of the pan, cover pan with a lid and cook until the top is set.

12) Remove pan from the stove and slide the eggs from the pan onto a plate.
13) Quarter them and leave them to cool slightly to ensure that they are not too hot to hold.
14) Use two of the quarters as a base for the "sandwich" and place ½ of the bacon slices on top of each.
15) Use the remaining quarters to complete the sandwich

Zucchini Parmesan Frittata (serves 4-6)

Ingredients

- 8 small, washed, but unpeeled zucchini
- 3 tablespoons coconut
- 2 tablespoons grass-fed butter
- 8 organic eggs
- 1/2 teaspoon freshly ground black pepper
- 1/2 cup grated, dairy free and home-made parmesan cheese substitute
- 1 teaspoon sea salt

Method

1) Cut zucchini into thin slices
2) Mix butter and oil and heat in a double-based pan and fry zucchini slowly until just tender.
3) Sprinkle both the pepper and the salt over the eggs and beat briskly.
4) Gently pour salted eggs over the zucchini.
5) Ensure temperature is on medium and cook frittata until just set.
6) Pepper the grated cheese on frittata top and broil slightly to brown lightly.
7) Allow to stand for a short while before cutting as desired.
8) Serve.

Slow Cooked Egg and Sausage Breakfast Casserole (serves 6)

Ingredients

- 1 medium head broccoli, chopped
- 12 ounces chicken sausages, cooked and sliced
- 1 cup shredded non-dairy cheddar cheese substitute (home-made)
- 10 organic eggs
- ¾ cup non-dairy whipped cream (home-made)
- 2 garlic cloves, minced
- ½ teaspoon salt and ¼ teaspoon pepper

Method

1) Grease the sides and base of your slow cooker well
2) Create a layer using half the broccoli, a second layer using half the sausage and yet another using half the cheese into the pot.
3) Repeat the procedure in step 2 with the other halves.
4) Place the remaining ingredients in a medium sized mixing bowl and mix well.
5) Gently pour the mixture into the crock-pot on top of the other ingredients ensuring even distribution.
6) Cover the slow cooker and cook on high for 3-3½ hours and the edges are well browned and the center is set.
7) Remove from cooker and serve as desired.

Chia and Berries Breakfast Pudding (Serves 4)

Ingredients

- 1 ½ cups whole coconut milk
- 1 ½ cup almond milk
- ¾ cup chia seeds 2 Tablespoons no-alcohol vanilla
- 2 teaspoons cinnamon
- ¾ teaspoon nutmeg (optional)
- 2 cups fresh berries
- 1/4 cup finely chopped walnuts

Method

1) Place all of the ingredients except the walnuts into a large mixing cup or bowl
2) Stir well until everything is integrated.
3) Pour pudding base into 4 10-ounce small bowls.
4) Cover and refrigerate over-night, this allows the pudding become creamy and to set.
5) To serve; top each bowl with ½ cup berries and 1 tablespoon of chopped walnuts.

Basic Chestnut Flour Crepes (makes 8 – 10)

Ingredients

- 7 ounces chestnut flour
- 1 cup coconut milk
- 1 cup tepid water
- 1 organic egg
- 1 tablespoon plus 1 teaspoon coconut oil

Method

1) Put coconut milk, egg and water in a food processor.
2) Measure out the chestnut flour and add to the blender.
3) Make a well in the center of the flour and pour the oil.
4) Blend the ingredients for 10 seconds and scrape any deposits from the sides blending jar then continue blending for an additional 8 seconds. Set batter aside.
5) Heat a large thick base frying pan over high heat and base with the teaspoon of oil.
6) Pour 1/3 cup of the batter into the pan and churn the batter around the pan base. Let the crepe cook until its surface appears dry.
7) Gently lift up an edge to check if the underside is golden brown.
8) If it is, carefully toss the crepe upside down and cook the other side until golden brown as well.

Spinach and Kale Eggs Florentine (Serves 2)

Ingredients

- 4 roughly chopped cups of spinach
- 4 roughly chopped of cups kale
- 2 minced cloves of garlic
- 1 tablespoon olive oil
- Pepper and sea salt for seasoning
- pinch of nutmeg
- 4 organic eggs

For Hollandaise sauce

- ½ cup clarified butter
- 2 organic egg yolks
- Juice from a small lemon

Method

1) Heat oil in a thick base pan over medium heat.
2) Add and fry garlic until slightly browned.
3) Add kale and spinach and stir here and there as the greens begin to shrivel.
4) Add salt, nutmeg and pepper to taste.
5) When the greens have shriveled enough, remove from the stove and set aside for use later on.
6) To make Hollandaise sauce, put half the butter and all the other ingredients into a double boiler over gently boiling water.
7) Briskly whisk the contents continuously until the butter is fully melted, to prevent curdling.

8) Add the remainder of the butter in small pieces and continue whisking until sauce thickens.

9) If curdling starts, remove from heat and add in a tablespoon of homemade coconut milk or any other nut milk cream.

10) Poach the eggs by using your best poaching method or the directions provided with your poacher.

11) Place a heap of greens on each serving plate, follow this by placing two poached eggs in each plate then lastly top with the Hollandaise Sauce.

12) You can add a dusting of paprika to garnish, if so desired.

Kale and Eggs (serves 2)

Ingredients

- 2 small bunches of kale
- 2 large orange bell peppers
- 1 brown or sweet onion
- 4 garlic cloves, finely chopped
- 2 tablespoons olive oil
- ¼ teaspoon sea salt
- ¼ teaspoon ground black pepper
- 8 large organic eggs
- Ingredients for sauce:
- ½ cup homemade mayonnaise
- 2 tablespoons Dijon mustard
- 1 teaspoon finely chopped fresh tarragon leaves

Method

1) Prepare kale by cutting the stem out with a sharp knife.
2) When ready, chop the leaves crosswise into ribbons.
3) Remove the top off of the peppers and cut them in quarters, top to bottom.
4) Remove the white membrane and deseed.
5) Slice the quarters again to make very thin strips.
6) Peel and cut the onion in half from top to root then slice the halves into thin half rings.
7) Heat the oil in a large stir-fry pan over medium heat then add the onion and the peppers.
8) Fry, stirring all the time, until vegetables are soft; should take about 4 minutes.
9) Add garlic and cook for 30 seconds more, continuously stirring.

10) Season with the salt and pepper.
11) Add the kale ribbons and mix, turn the leaves over to combine with the onions and peppers, ensure kale is thoroughly drenched in the oil and juices.
12) Cook the vegetables until the kale softens and shrinks in size, in 5-6 minutes or so.
13) Put lid on the pan and turn off the heat.
14) Keep the vegetables warm as the eggs get poached.
15) Make the sauce by whisking together the mayonnaise, mustard and tarragon leaves.
16) Arrange on serving dish when everything is ready.

Chia Breakfast Bowl

Ingredients

- 3 teaspoons Chia Seed
- 1 cup macadamia nut milk
- 1 teaspoon raw walnuts
- 1 teaspoon raw organic honey
- 1/3 cup frozen mixed berries

Method

1) Place all the ingredients save for the berries, in an airtight container and ensure they are thoroughly mixed.
2) Let mixture sit for 15 minutes, stir, then put container cover on and refrigerate, preferably overnight.
3) Serve with frozen berries.

Lunch Recipes

Mango and Grilled Shrimp Salad (serves 2 – 4)

Ingredients

<u>Shrimp Skewers</u>
- 1 pound peeled shrimp
- 2 roughly chopped red bell peppers
- Virgin olive oil

<u>Marinade</u>

- 1/4 cup lemon juice
- 1 pressed garlic clove
- 1/4 teaspoon red pepper flakes
- Sea salt and pepper to taste

<u>Mango Vinaigrette</u>

- 1/2 cup diced mango
- 2 tablespoons each of fresh orange juice and rice wine vinegar
- 1 tablespoon avocado oil
- A dash apart of sea salt and pepper

<u>Salad Ingredients</u>

- 2 cups chopped mango
- 2 diced avocados
- 1/2 cup diced red onion

- 8 cups personal choice salad greens

Method

1) To prepare the marinade, mix the ingredients; then place the mixture together with the shrimp into a plastic bag or container.
2) Put in refrigerator and leave for about 10 minutes, or just to give you time to prepare the vinaigrette
3) To make the vinaigrette; mix the given ingredients and stir to thoroughly mix.
4) Prepare the skewers by alternating the chopped peppers and the shrimp, thereafter, drizzle olive oil on each.
5) Switch grill to medium, place skewers in the grill and grill for between 4 and 5 minutes. Shrimp should pink to indicate doneness.
6) Prepare salad by topping with the shrimp skewers then drizzling vinaigrette as desired.

Fried Hake and Lentils

Ingredients

- 19 ounces hake fillets
- 5 ounces thinly sliced veal steak, cut into small pieces
- 4 spring onions, chopped
- 1 cup baby spinach, chopped
- 2 tablespoons coconut flour
- ½ teaspoon of sea salt
- 3 tablespoons high oleic safflower oil
- 1 garlic clove, crushed
- Juice of ½ a lemon
- A little grain-fed butter
- 14 ounces cooked lentils

Method

1) Sift together flour and salt and use the mixture to coat each fillet lightly before setting fillets aside.
2) Heat half the safflower oil its smoky then stir-fry the steak-lets until it's crispy.
3) Mix in both the garlic and the garlic and fry with the steak for a minute.
4) Add the lemon juice and the lentils then add seasoning to taste.
5) Add in the spinach and let it wilt slightly in the cooking temperature.
6) As spinach wilts, use a separate pan to heat the remaining safflower oil.
7) Add the grass-fed butter and fry each fillet side for about 3 minutes, avoid crowding them in the frying pan during frying.

8) When all fillets are fried, serve with the lentil salad.

Chicken and Vegetable Stew

Ingredients

- 12 ounces g chopped chicken breasts
- 2 tablespoons virgin olive oil
- 1 small sweet potato, peeled and chopped
- 2 carrots, sliced
- 2 ribs of celery, thinly sliced
- 1 bay leaf
- A chopped onion
- 2 thyme sprigs
- 1 peeled and minced clove of garlic
- 1 turnip, peeled and cut into small pieces
- ¾ teaspoon sea salt
- ¼ cup white wine vinegar
- 1 tablespoon arrowroot flour
- ¼ teaspoon ground pepper
- 4 cups chicken broth

Method

1) Heat olive oil slightly in a large pan over medium heat
2) Add in carrots, onions, garlic and celery and allow to gently cook until all soften.
3) Increase stove temperature to high before adding the chicken, the pepper and salt. Continuously stir the mixture.
4) Pour in the broth and stir in the sweet potato, turnip, bay leaf and thyme and cook.
5) Lower the temperature and let the mixture simmer to get the vegetables well cooked.

6) Briskly mix together the vinegar and the flour and pour into the chicken stew.
7) Stir frequently as stew cooks, until the stew thickens.
8) Remove from heat and serve with a salad.

Cauliflower and Carrot Salad

Ingredients

- 1 small head of cauliflower
- 1 pound carrot, peeled and finely grated
- ¼ cup chopped fresh coriander
- 1 tablespoon rapeseed oil
- 1 teaspoon olive oil
- ½ teaspoon mustard seeds
- 2 tablespoons sesame seeds
- 1 tablespoon cumin seeds
- Juice and zest of 1 lime

Method

1) Heat a thick base frying pan; add the mustard seeds and dry roast for ½ a minute.
2) Mix in the cumin seeds and allow to roast, when the mustard seeds begin popping, put seeds in a bowl to cool.
3) Use the same pan to toast the sesame seeds and set these aside also.
4) Break the cauliflower into florets and mix florets with grated carrot.
5) Heat the rapeseed oil slightly then add and stir-fry the cauliflower onion mixture for 5 minutes and remove from pan.
6) Mix cauliflower with the spices in a large bowl.
7) Add the coriander then drizzle with the olive oil and lime.
8) Top it all by sprinkling the sesame seeds.

Spiced Lentil Soup with Coconut (serves 4 – 6)

Ingredients

- 1 1/2 cup rinsed green lentils
- 4 cups vegetable broth
- 1 1/2 teaspoons turmeric
- 2 teaspoons dried thyme
- 1 tablespoon macadamia oil
- 1 diced, large onion
- 2 lemongrass stalks
- 1 teaspoon sea salt, a bit more if desired
- 1/2 teaspoon cardamom
- 1/2 teaspoon cinnamon
- A little red pepper flakes
- A pinch of grated fresh nutmeg
- 1 1/4 cup hemp milk
- Juice of a medium sized lemon
- 2 cups of chopped spinach
- 1 cup toasted flakes of coconut

Method

1) Place the lentils, turmeric, vegetable broth, and thyme into a large saucepan over medium heat.
2) Bring mixture to the boil then reduce heat to allow mixture to simmer for 20 minutes or so.
3) As lentils get cooked, slightly heat the macadamia oil in a pan (overheating burns macadamia oil).
4) Add the onion and stir-fry until slightly browned.
5) Add the finely minced lemongrass, cinnamon, salt, nutmeg, cardamom and the red pepper flakes and stir-fry for an additional minute.

6) Stir the onion mixture into the lentils and maintain the heat on low to simmer properly.
7) Add the hemp milk and greens then simmer for an additional five minutes, ensuring that you stir occasionally.
8) Taste for seasoning and add more if preferred then add the lemon juice.
9) Top with the coconut flakes and serve.

Slow Cooker Jambalaya (2-3 servings)

Ingredients

- 10 ounces cooked prawns
- 1 cup chopped onion
- 1 cup chopped green pepper
- 1 cup chopped celery
- 2 garlic cloves, minced
- 25 ounces diced tomatoes
- 2 cups turkey sausage or smoked sausage
- ¼ teaspoon each of hot sauce and pepper
- ½ teaspoon each of salt and dried thyme
- 1 tablespoon dried parsley

Method

1) Add all ingredients except prawns and stir well
2) Cook on high for 3-4 hours
3) Add prawns to crock-pot for the last 15 minutes of cooking time.

Crock Pot Chili Beef (serves 4)

Ingredients

- 1 pound lean beef, ground, browned and drained
- 3 stalks celery, diced
- 1 cup onion, chopped
- 2 cloves garlic, mince
- 11 ounces diced tomato with juice
- 1 pound home-made tomato sauce
- 11 ounces low sodium beef broth
- 1 cup hot water
- 1½ teaspoon chili powder
- ½ teaspoon each of cumin, oregano and paprika
- Dash of cayenne pepper
- 1 teaspoon each of salt and black pepper

Method

1) Mix all the ingredients in the crock pot
2) Cook on low heat for 6-8 hours

Cheesy Cauliflower Soup (serves 4)

This is one of the most weight loss friendly soups you can ever have. It has only 6 calories per serving which will ensure that you certainly head in the right weight loss direction.

Ingredients

- 1 cauliflower head, chopped
- 1 stalk celery, chopped
- ½ teaspoon Worcestershire sauce (home-made)
- 4 cups chicken stock
- 1 cup heavy coconut milk cream
- 2 cups American cheese vegan substitute, shredded
- Chopped chives
- 1 onion, chopped
- Salt and pepper to taste.

Method

1) Put cauliflower, onion, celery and stock in a crock pot
2) Cover and cook on low for 6-8 hours
3) Puree the mixture and return to pot
4) Add cream, Worcestershire sauce, cheese, salt and pepper to the mixture and stir to mix
5) Turn heat to high and cook until hot and melted then serve hot.

Roasted Beet and Carrot Salad

Ingredients

- 1 medium size garlic head
- Sea salt for seasoning
- 1 small bunch of peeled carrots
- 1 small bunch of scrubbed beets, greens trimmed
- Pepper for seasoning
- 1 small bunch of rainbow chard
- Juice from a small lemon
- 4 tablespoons of virgin olive oil
- 1/3 cup hulled pepitas, raw

Method

1) Preheat the oven to 150° C.
2) Place a large saucepan half full of water on the stove and allow to boil.
3) Cut and remove the woody bottom of the garlic head, enough to reveal the clove bottoms.
4) Prepare a foil paper; sprinkle a teaspoon of olive oil and a little sea salt.
5) Roll the garlic head in olive oil and wrap the foil paper around it and place in an ovenproof dish. Place dish into the oven.
6) Bake for about 15 minutes and then remove from oven and allow to cool. Increase the oven temperature to 200°C.
7) Place the carrots in a bowl of boiling water for 2 minutes to blanch; then allow time to cool. Put beets in a small saucepan with the same water used for the carrots and boil for 8 – 10 minutes.

8) Remove saucepan from heat remove and run beets under cold water to ensure the skins readily peel off. Use your fingers to peel off skin, or a peeler if skin appears tougher.

9) Cut the carrots into halves and the beets into quarters or sixths, let size determine. Arrange them on baking sheets separate from each other, then drizzle each vegetable with 1 teaspoon of olive oil and sprinkle a little sea salt.

10) Place trays into the oven to roast for 15 – 20 minutes, flip the vegetables halfway through the set time.

11) Arrange the chard on another baking sheet and drizzle just a little oil. Additionally rub oil all over the leaves and add a pinch of sea salt.

12) Bake the leaves for 5 or 6 minutes, or just allow leaves to soften and brown slightly without getting burnt.

13) In the meantime, make the dressing by squeezing the roasted and then cooled garlic out of its skin. Put into a small bowl, and gently mash with a fork.

14) Put lemon juice and a pinch of sea salt then mix well.

15) When well mixed, whisk in a tablespoon of olive oil and keep up until mixture emulsifies.

16) Toast the pepitas by heating a medium skillet over medium heat and adding a little olive oil together with the pepitas.

17) Fry for 1-2 minutes while stirring constantly. When the pepitas begin to pop, remove from heat and toss with a little salt. Allow to cool.

18) Toss beets and the carrots with the dressing to serve. Arrange roasted chard on the first in a serving plate, then top with carrots and beets. Finally, drizzle a little more of the dressing and toasted pepitas.

19) Season as desired and serve.

Buttered Rasher-Wrapped Sausages (4 servings)

Ingredients

- 8 thin veal rashers
- 8 grass-fed-beef sausages
- 12 sage leaves
- 2 tablespoons suet
- 2 tablespoons butter (grass-fed)
- 6 ounces roughly torn soft spinach leaves
- 2 red onions sliced
- Sea salt and ground black pepper

Method

1) Preheat the oven to 220°C.
2) Place a rasher around each sausage before gently arranging them in a roasting pan.
3) Add the onions and sage leaves then spoon over the suet making sure to be generous over the onions.
4) Place on middle rack in the oven and roast for 30–40 minutes
5) Heat butter in a thick based pan over medium heat then add the spinach; stir-fry until just wilted.
6) Serve sausages and with stir-fried spinach on the side.

Spicy Steak Bites (serves 4)

Ingredients

- 25 ounces cubed chuck steak
- 3 chopped onions
- 6 coarsely chopped cloves of garlic
- 1 ½ tablespoons of peeled then grated ginger
- 1 ½ cups of home-made coconut cream
- 1 tablespoon each, of ground cumin and cinnamon
- 2 teaspoons ground coriander
- 1 ½ teaspoons ground turmeric
- ½ teaspoon ground cloves of garlic
- 2 teaspoons olive oil
- 1 teaspoon chili powder
- 2 deseeded and chopped red chilies
- 2 large strips of lemon rind with as much of the pith as possible removed
- Sea salt for seasoning

Method

1) Put all the ingredients except meat, chilies, lemon rind and in half the coconut cream, in a blender and pulse into a paste.
2) Heat olive oil in a thick bottomed saucepan and fry the paste until it turns slightly dark in color.
3) Add the cubed steaks, the red chilies, remaining coconut cream, lemon-rind and salt; and gently bring to the boil.
4) Reduce the heat and allow to simmer gently for about an hour and a half.
5) Check to see if the meat is tender enough before adding 3 teaspoons of lemon juice.

6) Allow a couple of minutes for a thorough combination of all ingredients.
7) Serve and enjoy.

Baked Beef Curry (serves 2-3)

Ingredients

- 1 tablespoon suet
- 17 ounces beef mince
- 1 chopped onion
- 3 crushed cloves of garlic
- 4 finely sliced celery sticks
- 1 tablespoon tomato paste
- 2 cups homemade beef stock
- 7 ounces extra fine green beans, thinly sliced
- Sea salt and black pepper
- 17 ounces cauliflower florets
- 1 cup homemade chicken stock
- 2 tablespoons grass-fed butter
- 2 teaspoons finely chopped fresh thyme

Method

1) Melt the suet in a thick-bottom saucepan under medium-hot heat.
2) Put the mince into the pan and cook until well browned.
3) Add the garlic, onion, garlic, tomato paste, celery; and beef stock and stir gently to mix.
4) Reduce heat to medium and cook for 25–30 minutes.
5) When the mixture is cooked, stir in the green beans and season to your liking.
6) Transfer to an ovenproof dish.
7) Preheat oven to 200ºC.
8) Cook together the cauliflower, chicken stock and half the butter in a pot until cauliflower is soft.

9) Pulp the mixture until as smooth as possible before stirring in the thyme.
10) Season well and spread over the mince mixture.
11) Break remaining butter into the smallest possible pieces and evenly top the mixture.
12) Cut into sizable pieces and bake for 18-20 minutes or until golden.
13) Serve and enjoy.

Brussels Sprout Chips (serves 2)

Ingredients

- 2 cups of Brussels sprouts leaves
- 1½ tablespoons high macadamia oil
- Mixed spices
- Sea salt

Method

1) Preheat oven to 210°C
2) Combine the Brussels sprouts leaves with the oil, salt and spice; then mix well.
3) Line a baking tray with an anti-stick baking sheet and arrange leaves in single layer on the sheet.
4) Place baking tray into the oven and bake until the leaves are crispy and slightly browned in the edges
5) Serve as hot as possible.

Curried Cabbage and Broccoli

Ingredients

- 4 tablespoons coconut oil
- 1 chopped onion
- 1 fresh ginger, chopped
- 1 teaspoon ground turmeric
- 2 tablespoons curry powder
- 2 green chilies, chopped
- 1 cup canned tomato
- 1 large cabbage, shredded
- 2 cups each broccoli florets and chopped carrots
- Handful chopped coriander

Method

1) Heat the coconut oil in a frying pan
2) Add and fry onions until soft
3) Add all the remaining ingredients except coriander
4) Reduce heat and cook covered for 10 minutes
5) Add coriander just before serving

Cabbage and Mushroom Stroganoff (serves 4 – 6)

Ingredients

- 4 tablespoons oil
- 1 large onion, chopped
- 2 tablespoons paprika
- 4 pounds sliced mushrooms
- 1 white and 1 red cabbages, shredded
- 3½ cups vegetable stock
- 8.45 fluid ounces non-dairy double whipped cream
- Sea salt and pepper

Method

1) Heat oil in a large frying pan
2) Add onions and fry until soft
3) Add paprika, cabbage and mushrooms and cook for 3 minutes
4) Add stock and simmer covered, for 8 minutes
5) Add the cream and season well then cook for a further 4 minutes before serving

Low Carb Crock Pot Chili (serves 4)

Ingredients

- 1 pound lean beef, ground, browned and drained
- 3 stalks celery, diced
- 1 cup onion, chopped
- 2 cloves garlic, minced
- 11 ounces diced tomato with juice
- 1 pound home-made tomato sauce
- 1 ½ cups low sodium beef broth
- 1 cup hot water
- 1½ teaspoon chili powder
- ½ teaspoon each of cumin, oregano and paprika
- Dash of cayenne pepper
- 1 teaspoon each of salt and black pepper

Method

1) Mix all the ingredients in the crock pot
2) Cook on low heat for 6-8 hours

Parmesan Cauliflower Soup (serves 4)

This is one of the most weight loss friendly soups you can ever have. It has only 6 calories per serving which will ensure that you certainly head in the right weight loss direction.

Ingredients

- 1 cauliflower head, chopped
- 1 stalk celery, chopped
- ½ teaspoon Worcestershire sauce (home-made)
- 4 cups chicken stock
- 1 cup heavy coconut milk cream
- 2 cups parmesan cheese vegan substitute, shredded
- Chopped chives
- 1 onion, chopped
- Salt and pepper to taste.

Method

1) Put cauliflower, onion, celery and stock in a crock pot
2) Cover and cook on low for 6-8 hours
3) Puree the mixture and return to pot
4) Add cream, Worcestershire sauce, cheese, salt and pepper to the mixture and stir to mix
5) Turn heat to high and cook until hot and melted
6) Serve and enjoy.

Teriyaki Fried Brown Lentils with Chicken (4 servings)

Ingredients

- 22 ounces chicken breasts
- 2 tablespoons rapeseed oil
- 2 chopped onions
- 1 medium julienned carrot
- 1 large beaten egg
- 2 cups cold boiled lentils
- 2 tablespoons roasted garlic and home-made teriyaki sauce mixture
- a teaspoon of chili paste

Method

1) Thinly slice chicken into strips.
2) Heat rapeseed oil in large thick based pot over high heat.
3) Add chicken, carrot, onions, and chili sauce to the pot and stir-fry until chicken is cooked through.
4) Stir in the egg and continuously stir gently until mixture firms.
5) Add lentils, stirring all the time and cook until thoroughly heated.
6) Add teriyaki and ginger sauce before removing from heat; mix well and serve.

Cauliflower Tabbouler (serves 3)

Ingredients

- 1 de-stemmed and chopped cauliflower head
- 11 ounces halved cherry tomatoes
- 1 1/2 cups chopped fresh parsley
- 1/2 cup chopped cilantro
- 4 finely chopped stalks of celery
- 2 thinly sliced green onions
- Sea salt and pepper for seasoning

<u>Dressing</u>

- 1/3 cup good quality virgin olive oil
- 2 tablespoons red wine vinegar
- 2 tablespoons cranberry syrup
- Pinch of sea salt

Method

1) Place and pulse the cauliflower in a food processor until it looks like the grains of rice.
2) Remove from processor and put into a mixing bowl.
3) Scrape down the bowl sides if some of the cauliflower attaches to the sides.
4) Add the green onions, parsley, tomatoes, cilantro and celery into the bowl.
5) Separately stir the dressing ingredients in a different bowl and mix well before you pour and mix dressing with the cauliflower mixture.
6) Stir well to combine thoroughly. Add more salt and pepper if desired.

7) Place in the fridge and allow to stand for between 30 and 40 minutes before serving.

Creamy Chicken and Peppers Enchilada
(serves 4)

Ingredients

- 2 tablespoons of high oleic safflower oil
- 9 ounces diced mushrooms
- 1 chopped red onion
- 1 chopped garlic clove
- 1 each of deseeded and chopped orange and yellow bell peppers
- 4 deboned and skinless organic chicken fillets
- 15 ounces roughly cut tomatoes
- ½ cup salt-less chicken stock
- ¼ teaspoon dried red chili flakes
- peel of 1 small lemon
- 3 dried bay leaves
- 4 each of fresh thyme and oregano stems
- Freshly ground black pepper and salt to season
- chunks of home-made non-dairy hard cheese

Method

1) Use a deep saucepan to heat 1 tablespoon of high oleic safflower oil.
2) Add the mushrooms and stir-fry on a high heat for 5 minutes.
3) When well browned, add salt and pepper to season.

4) Place the mushrooms in a separate container.
5) Using the same pan, add the onion and fry over moderate heat until translucent.
6) Add the garlic and sweet peppers into the pan and cook for a couple of minutes more.
7) Season the chicken fillets on both sides with salt and the black pepper.
8) Transfer the vegetables a different container and brown the fillets on both sides using the same pan.
9) Add the all the remaining ingredients and a little water and cook for about three minutes.
10) Add the mushrooms then cover pan and allow to boil on very low heat, for roughly 20 minutes.
11) Crumble the cheese on top and leave until the top turns golden.

Slow Cooker Thai Beef with Roasted Cauliflower (serves 4)

Ingredients

- 4 teaspoons red/ green Thai curry paste
- 1 $^2/_3$ cups organic coconut milk
- 3 tablespoons fish sauce
- 2 pounds steak or chuck roast in sizable pieces
- 9 ounces mushrooms
- Medium onion and carrot both sliced thinly
- 11 ounces cauliflower florets
- 2 teaspoons salt
- ½ teaspoon pepper
- 11 ½ ounces trimmed fresh green beans

Method

1) Whisk the paste, milk and sauce in the slow cooker.
2) Add the remaining ingredients except beans and stir to ensure sauce coats everything
3) Add the beans but do not mix
4) Cook on low heat for 8 hours, in the last 30 minutes, stir in the beans at ten minute intervals.
5) Serve with roasted cauliflower

Sun-Dried Tomato Turkey and Dried Tomato Burgers with Avocado
(serves 4)

Ingredients

- 20 ounces of dark ground turkey
- 2 tablespoons finely chopped fresh parsley
- 12 large, chopped, sundried tomatoes
- 1 tablespoon and 1 teaspoon Dijon mustard
- ¼ teaspoon of sea salt
- 2 pinches red pepper flakes (optional)
- 1 teaspoon olive oil
- ¼ teaspoon ground black pepper
- 1 peeled, deseeded and mashed avocado
- 1 teaspoon lemon juice
- 2 pinches sea salt

Method

1) Mix the ground turkey, chopped herbs, dried tomatoes, peppers, mustard and salt until smoothly combined.
2) Work the burger mixture with your hands to ensure thorough mixing.
3) Divide burger mixture into 4 equal portions and shape into rounded patties or shape as desired, but make them ¾ inches thick to cook easily.
4) You can use a ring mold if you want to shape them round and perfect.
5) Place oil in a thick base pan and heat it over medium low temperature. When the oil is slightly hot, add the patties and fry until a nice browned crust develops, in between 3 and 4 minutes.

6) Turn the patties over and put the lid back on the pan. Reduce the temperature to low and cook burgers for between 7 and 8 minutes, in which time they should reach an internal temperature of 85°C and the meat is pink no more.
7) As the patties are cooking, put the avocado, lemon juice, mayonnaise and salt into a food processor and puree until creamy and smooth.
8) Serve burgers with a quarter of the avocado cream on top.

Chicken Dijonnaise (4 servings)

- 2 chicken breasts, skin removed
- 1/8 cup Dijon mustard
- 1/8 cup mayonnaise (Dr. Hyman's)
- Juice from a small fresh lemon
- ¼ cup virgin olive oil
- A teaspoon of sea salt
- 1/2 teaspoon of pepper

Method

1) Preheat oven to 175° C
2) Cut breasts in half to have four pieces.
3) Place the four pieces of chicken in a lightly greased baking tray.
4) In a small mixing bowl, thoroughly mix the mustard and the mayonnaise
5) Place the olive oil, lemon juice, salt, pepper and salt and lightly mix together.
6) Mix in the blend of mayonnaise and mustard and ensure they are thoroughly combined.
7) Carefully pour mixture over the pieces of chicken ensuring they are fully covered.
8) Place and bake in the heated oven for between 30 and 35 minutes or until the chicken juices run clear and chicken starts browning.
9) Remove from oven and serve as desired.

Baked Garlic and Cheese Chicken (serves 6)

Ingredients

- 6 chicken breasts
- 7 ounces grated non-dairy home-made hard cheese
- 2 teaspoons crushed garlic
- 2 tablespoons hemp flour
- ¼ cup grass-fed butter
- ¼ teaspoon sea salt
- Juice from a small lemon

Method

1) Preheat oven to 175 º C.
2) Lightly grease a biggish baking tray and put the pieces of chicken.
3) Thoroughly mix together the garlic, flour, butter, salt, and lemon juice.
4) Evenly brush the mixture over the chicken breasts.
5) Place in the heated oven and bake for 50 - 60 minutes or until when chicken is tender.
6) Remove from oven and sprinkle the cheese.
7) Put tray back into the oven and bake for 5 minutes, cheese should have melted.
8) Serve as desired.

Oven Baked Rabbit Dijon

Ingredients

- 1¾ pounds rabbit meat
- 2 tablespoons Dijon mustard
- 3 tablespoons rapeseed oil
- ½ cup wine vinegar
- Juice of half an orange
- ¼ teaspoon sea salt
- 2 medium sized onions, chopped
- $1^1/_2$ ounces very thinly sliced steak.
- Pepper to season

Method

1) Preheat the oven to 175 ° C
2) Cut the rabbit into pieces and sprinkle pepper and salt, thereafter; spread the mustard on the pieces.
3) Grease a baking dish and place rabbit pieces then drizzle first the oil, then the vinegar around it.
4) Cut steak into ½ inch pieces; mix with the onions and pepper these on top of rabbit pieces.
5) Cover dish and bake for between 25 and 35 minutes.
6) Remove dish from oven, turn the pieces over and drizzle the orange juice over them.
7) Place back into the oven and bake uncovered for 30 minutes more, meat should be tender after that.
8) Serve as desired.

Spiced Salmon with Chili Sauce (4 servings)

With only 325 calories per serving, this dish is a sure way of enjoying good food while losing weight.

Ingredients

- 4 x 7 ounces salmon fillets
- 2 teaspoon chili sauce
- 1 teaspoon honey
- ¼ teaspoon each of ground red pepper, ground turmeric and salt
- $^1/_8$ teaspoon garlic powder

Method

1) Preheat cooking spray coated broiler
2) Combine all ingredients except the fish in a bowl and stir with a fork.
3) Rub mixture evenly over fish
4) Place fillets on broiler, skin-side down
5) Broil for 8-10 minutes
6) Remove from stove and serve.

Cabbage Roll Stew (4 servings)

Ingredients

- 1 pound lean ground beef
- 1 medium onion, choppe
- 1 ½ pounds stewed tomatoes
- 17 ounces home-made tomato sauce
- 1 tablespoon minced garlic
- 1 cup chicken broth
- 1 teaspoon grated green pepper
- ½ teaspoon hot pepper
- ½ cabbage head, chopped

Method

1) Fry beef and onions in a pot until browned.
2) Place all remaining ingredients except cabbage in a slow cooker and mix well.
3) Add beef mixture followed by cabbage and cook on low for 5-6 hours

Lamb and Mushrooms (serves 3 – 4)

Ingredients

- 1 pound lamb steak, thinly sliced across the grain into ½cm thick pieces
- 2 cm long chunk fresh ginger, chopped
- 12 spring greens, sliced
- 6 ounces pack sliced mushrooms
- 4 tablespoons vegan oyster sauce (home-made)
- 2 tablespoon high oleic safflower oil

Method

1) Heat a deep skillet until smoking hot, add 1 tsp. oil; stir-fry the meat until browned all over. Remove meat and wipe skillet
2) Add a little more oil. Stir-fry the ginger until golden,
3) Add greens and mushrooms. Stir and cook for 3 minutes or so.
4) Add the steak and sauce, mix. Cook for 3 more minutes until sauce thickens a little and everything is thoroughly warmed.
5) Remove from stove and serve with a salad.

Beef and Veggie Stuffed Peppers (Serves 4)

Ingredients

- 4 large orange bell peppers
- 2 tablespoons olive oil
- 1 pound grass-fed, ground beef
- 1 small yellow onion, chopped finely
- 4 cloves of garlic, finely chopped
- 1 Tablespoon plus 1 teaspoon ancho chili powder
- 2 teaspoons cumin
- 2 teaspoons paprika
- 2 teaspoons dried oregano
- ½ teaspoon sea salt
- 1 small zucchini, quartered lengthwise and chopped small
- 12 ounces diced tomatoes
- ¼ teaspoon ground black pepper
- ¼ cup chopped Italian parsley leaves

Method

1) Trim off any green stem on the top of each bell pepper.
2) Cut the pepper in half, from top to bottom.
3) Remove the seeds and white membrane to leave you with a cup of sorts to hold the filling. Set them aside while you make the filling.
4) In a large stir-fry pan, heat olive oil over medium heat.
5) Add onion and cook, stirring here and there, until the onion is soft and clear, should take about 3 minutes.
6) Turn the heat down to medium low if the onions cook too quickly.

7) Add the garlic, cumin, paprika, and oregano and cook 1-2 minutes.
8) Add the zucchini and cook until it is softened, about 3-4 minutes.
9) Add the beef, and cook until the meat is no longer pink, breaking it up with a wooden spoon and stirring, about 8-10 minutes.
10) Preheat oven to 175°C.
11) Add the tomatoes to beef and simmer until the tomatoes have broken down and flavors have blended, about 8-10 minutes longer. Season with the salt, pepper and fold in the fresh herbs.
12) Divide filling between the 8 pepper halves.
13) Place stuffed peppers in a large casserole dish, cover with foil and bake in the oven for about 30 minutes or when the center of the filling is 85°C.
14) You can store the peppers refrigerated, covered before baking for 2-3 days. To bake, you just bring them back to room temperature and bake as indicated above.

Venison and Mushrooms

Ingredients

- 1 pound venison, cut into cubes, boiled for 1½ hours and dried
- 1 cm long chunk fresh ginger, chopped
- 12 ounces spring greens, sliced
- 6 ounces pack sliced mushrooms
- 4 tablespoon oyster sauce
- 2 tablespoon each red wine vinegar sauce and coconut oil

Method

1) Mix sauces and set aside.
2) Heat a deep skillet until smoking hot, add 1 tsp. oil; stir-fry the boiled meat until browned all over. Remove meat and wipe skillet
3) Add a little more oil. Stir-fry the ginger until golden,
4) Add greens and mushrooms. Stir and cook for 3
5) Add the venison and soy sauce mixture. Cook for 3 more minutes until sauce thickens a little and everything is thoroughly warmed.
6) Serve with a salad.

Fish and Baby Tomato Bake (4 servings)

Fish is a healthier substitute for other meat types and mostly has healthy fats and high quality proteins, both of which have health advantages for our bodies.

Ingredients

- 4-6 fish cutlets
- 1 tablespoon garlic and herb seasoning
- 4 ounces each of mixed baby tomatoes and steamed Brussels sprouts
- Garlic bulb, halved horizontally
- 3 tablespoons olive oil
- Sea salt and freshly ground pepper

Method

1) Preheat oven to 200 °C.
2) Grease an oven-proof dish
3) Season fish with garlic and herb seasoning and place in dish together with tomatoes, garlic and sprouts.
4) Drizzle with olive oil and season with salt and pepper
5) Bake for 15 minutes
6) Serve with a salad

Sautéed Minute Steaks (serves 4)

Steak is good for weight loss because it is low in fat and therefore contains fewer calories. And beef is generally high in protein, which is necessary for good health.

Ingredients

- ½ cup coconut or hemp flour
- 1 teaspoon garlic salt
- ½ teaspoon pepper
- 21 ounces beef steaks, cubed
- 2/3 cup home-made tomato sauce
- 2 tablespoons lemon juice
- 1½ teaspoons ground mustard

Method

1) Thoroughly mix flour, salt and pepper
2) Use mixture to coat steaks
3) Grease large skillet and cook steaks over low heat for 4 minutes on each side.
4) Remove from skillet
5) Stir in remaining ingredients until heated through
6) Serve with the salad

Broiled Tilapia Parmesan (serves 3 – 4)

Ingredients

- ¼ cup home-made vegan parmesan cheese
- 2 tablespoons each of grass-fed butter and Dr. M. Hyman's mayonnaise
- 1 tablespoon lemon juice
- $^1/_8$ teaspoon each of dried basil, celery salt and ground black pepper
- 1 small onion, grated
- 1 pound tilapia fillets

Method

1) Preheat broiler and spray no-stick spray
2) Mix all ingredients except fish in a bowl
3) Single layer the fillets on pan and broil a few inches from heat for 3 minutes
4) Flip and redo
5) Remove from oven and put cheese mixture on top side
6) Broil until topping is browned and fish flakes easily
7) Remove from heat and serve

Did you know?

Tilapia can help you maintain healthy blood pressure while keeping many diseases at bay because it is a good source of Omega 3 fatty acids.

Sweet Potato Fritters

Ingredients

- 14 ounces grated sweet potatoes
- 9 ounces chopped red or sweet onions
- ½ cup almond or coconut flour
- 1 beaten organic egg
- 1 teaspoon Chinese 5 spice
- Sea salt and pepper
- 2 tablespoon high oleic safflower oil

Method

1) Use a good size mixing bowl to combine all ingredients and mix thoroughly, leave out the oil.
2) Heat a double based frying pan over medium heat and add in the oil.
3) Spoon the mixture into the frying pan to make several fritters.
4) Gently put pressure on the spooned mixtures while in the pan.
5) Fry fritters until crusty and well browned on one side; turn and repeat to crust and brown the other side.
6) Remove from heat and serve as hot as desired.

Did you know?

Sweet potatoes are a highly versatile vegetable that you can roast, boil, bake, fry, roast, steam, puree, or grill.

Roasted Portobello Mushrooms (2 servings)

90% of mushrooms is water therefore they are a low calorie delicacy.

Ingredients

- 1 pound de-stemmed Portobello mushrooms
- 2 tablespoons macadamia oil
- ½ teaspoon ground black pepper
- Moroccan spice rub
- Sea salt

Method

1) Preheat oven to 200°C
2) Place the mushrooms, macadamia oil, Moroccan spice rub, sea salt and black pepper in a bowl and toss until thoroughly combined.
3) Line a baking tray and nicely arrange the mushrooms stem-side facing down.
4) Place in oven and roast for about 7 minutes or until the visible part is brown.
5) Turn the mushrooms and roast for 7-10 more minutes.
6) Season to desired taste and serve.

Butternut Cups

Ingredients

- Butternuts
- Flaked salmon or tuna
- 1 tablespoon grass-fed butter

Method

1) Peel the butternut and remove the insides as well.
2) Boil the butternuts for about ten minutes but do not let them get too soft.
3) Remove from heat and stuff with the fish.
4) Spread the butter on top of the fish and steam the stuffed butternuts for 15-20 minutes or until the butter is fully melted.
5) Serve and enjoy.

Dinner Recipes

Cheesy Beef Cauliflower (Serves 2)

Ingredients

- 1 pound deboned beef sirloin
- 2 cups cauliflower florets
- 4 cups broccoli florets
- 4 tablespoons roughly torn non-dairy hard home-made cheese
- 2-3 tablespoons olive oil
- Salt and freshly ground black pepper

Method

1) Cube the beef into bite sized pieces and add seasoning
2) First place a layer of the vegetables in a slow cooker
3) Place the meat atop the vegies and add the rest at the sides and on the meat.
4) Add the water and allow to cook on medium heat for 4 to five hours
5) After it's cooked, dust with the cheese on top and serve

Slow Cooked Tilapia Cheese (serves 4)

Ingredients

- 2 pounds tilapia
- 2 ounces hard organic home-made cheese substitute
- ¼ cup grass-fed butter
- 3 tablespoons Dr. M Hyman's home-made mayonnaise
- ¼ teaspoon garlic powder
- A small onion, chopped
- Salt and ¼ teaspoon of black pepper, preferably freshly ground

Method

1) Spray non-stick spray or use any other anti-stick product at the base and sides of the slow cooke
2) Gently place the fish into the cooker and add a dash of seasoning on top.
3) Separately combine garlic, butter, pepper, onion, salt and mayonnaise until thoroughly mixed then spoon mixture on top of the tilapia.
4) Cook on medium heat for 2 hours thirty minutes.
5) Sprinkle the cheese evenly on top, reduce heat to low and cook for an hour more.
6) Serve and enjoy.

Chili Chicken with Mushroom (Servings: 4)

Ingredients

- 2 tablespoons of olive oil
- 9 ounces diced mushrooms
- 1 chopped red onion
- 1 chopped garlic clove
- 1 each of deseeded and chopped orange and yellow peppers
- 4 deboned and skinless organic chicken fillets
- 14 ounces roughly cut tomatoes
- ½ cup salt-less chicken stock
- ½ teaspoon dried red chili flakes
- peel of 1 small lemon
- 3 dried bay leaves
- 4 each of fresh thyme and oregano stems
- Freshly ground black pepper and sea salt to season
- 2 teaspoons of grass-fed butter

Method

1) Use a deep saucepan to heat 1 tablespoon olive oil.
2) Add the mushrooms and stir-fry on a high heat for 5 minutes.
3) When well browned, add salt and pepper to season.
4) Place the mushrooms in a separate container.
5) Using the same pan, add the onion and fry over moderate heat until translucent.
6) Add the garlic and sweet peppers into the pan and cook for a couple of minutes more.
7) Season the chicken fillets on both sides with salt and the black pepper.

8) Transfer the vegetables a different container and brown the fillets on both sides using the same pan.
9) Add the all the remaining ingredients and a little water and cook for about three minutes.
10) Add the mushrooms then cover pan and allow to boil on very low heat, for roughly 20 minutes.
11) Dot the butter on top and leave until the top turns golden.

Sweet Potato Fish Cakes (serves 3 – 4)

Ingredients

- 1 pound hake or whiting steaks
- 2 medium sized sweet potatoes, boiled and mashed
- I onion, grated
- 3 tablespoons chopped flat leaf parsley
- Juice of a small lemon
- 2 beaten organic eggs
- 4 tablespoons coconut or hemp flour
- Sea salt and ground pepper

Method

1) Thoroughly grease a slow cooker
2) Place the fish into a blender and lightly blend
3) Place fish in a mixing bowl fish and add rest of ingredients.
4) Mix thoroughly then shape mixture into six cakes of roughly same size.
5) Place the cakes of a floured board and lightly roll
6) Place cakes individually into the slow cooker.
7) Place lid on and cook on medium heat for four to four and a half hours.
8) Remove from cooker, place on a greased baking tray and grill for 2 minutes or so before serving.

Did you know?

Eggs contain proteins, vitamin D and folic acid. These are believed to increase alertness. Lack of vitamin D is considered as one of the causes of depression and lowered mental functions.

Cauliflower Tabbouleh Salad(serves 4)

Ingredients

- 1 medium sized cauliflower, washed and dried
- ½ medium sized onion, chopped
- ½ cup flat leaf parsley
- ½ cup each of mint, dill and chives
- 5 ounces finely diced cucumber
- 1 medium tomato, finely diced
- juice of 1 small lemon
- 1 tablespoon olive oil
- salt and pepper
- 8 beef bangers

Method

1) Cut cauliflower into hunks and put in a food processor.
2) Blend until fine but not pureed then remove from processor and set aside.
3) Blend the onion, chives, parsley, dill and mint until fine.
4) Place into a mixing bowl and add the cauliflower mixture.
5) Add the cucumber, tomato, lemon juice and half the olive oil and mix well.
6) Season it to taste and set aside until ready to use.
7) Slightly heat the remaining olive oil in double base frying pan over medium heat.
8) Gently place the sausages and fry for 13-15 minutes, ensure they are cooked through before removal.
9) Serve with the salad.

Buttered Garlic Cauliflower Mash (serves 4)

Ingredients

- 1 medium head cauliflower - broken into florets
- 1/3 cup grated home-made, non-dairy, hard and preferably aged cheese
- 1 crushed clove of garlic
- 4 tablespoons grass-fed butter (best home-made)
- salt and pepper to taste
- sprinkle of nutmeg

Method

1) Dip the cauliflower florets in boiling salted water and continue boiling, for about 15 - 20 minutes.
2) When soft, drain, set the florets aside and discard the water.
3) Use the same pot to heat the butter and gently fry the garlic for 4-5 minutes.
4) Add the boiled florets and pulp with a vegetable masher until fine.
5) Add the grated cheese to the mashed mixture and mix well.
6) Season as desired and serve with a sprinkle of nutmeg.

Steak with Fried Tomatoes (serves 5 – 8)

Ingredients

- 3 pounds rib-eye steaks at room temperature
- 2 tablespoons olive oil
- 14 ounces cherry tomatoes
- 1 tablespoon chopped fresh rosemary needles
- 2 chopped cloves of garlic
- 2 tablespoons roughly chopped capers
- Sea salt
- ground black pepper
- 1 tablespoon each of grass-fed butter and chopped flat parsley
- zest of 1 lemon

Method

1) Heat large double base frying pan over medium heat and add the oil.
2) Fry the tomatoes in the oil until the skins rip open.
3) Add the capers, garlic and rosemary and cook together for five minutes.
4) Season with salt and pepper as desired, then stir in the butter and lemon zest, and cook for 2 more minutes.
5) Remove from heat, add the parsley and set aside until required.
6) Add seasoning to the steaks before frying them in a very hot frying. Ensure they maintain their warmth.
7) Warm the serving plates and add the steaks. Top steaks with reheated tomatoes and serve with a salad of choice.

Spiced Chicken Curry (serves 5)

Ingredients

- 18 ounces chicken pieces, with skin on
- Sea salt
- 4 tablespoons olive oil
- 3 chopped large onions
- 5 peeled and chopped tomatoes
- 2 tablespoons curry powder
- 1 chopped fresh green chili
- 1 teaspoon dried thyme
- ½ cup water
- chicken stock
- Pepper

Method

1) Use a thick based frying pan to slightly heat half the oil and use to fry the pieces of chicken until well browned. Gradually add salt as you fry.
2) Remove chicken from frying pan and place in a separate container.
3) Add the remaining oil and use to sauté the onions until they are soft and tender.
4) Add the tomatoes, chili, curry powder and thyme to the onions and mix well and allow to cook for 4-5 minutes.
5) Pour in the stock and water and stock allow to boil.
6) Gently place the chicken pieces into the pot with the onion mixture.
7) Ensure the heat is on low, then put the lid on and simmer for 40 minutes.
8) Season as desired and serve with a salad of choice.

Veal and Shallot Casserole with Sage and Mushrooms (serves 4)

Ingredients

- 2 tablespoons grape seed oil
- 2 teaspoons extra virgin olive oil
- 1 tablespoon grass-fed butter
- 14 ounces veal
- 2 teaspoons Dijon mustard
- 1 tsp. wholegrain mustard
- 4 shallots, peeled and chopped
- 1 chopped clove of garlic
- 9 ounces sliced Portobello mushrooms
- 3 ounces dried shiitake mushrooms
- 1 cup boiling water
- 7 roughly torn fresh sage leaves
- 3 tablespoons sherry
- ½ cup reserved mushroom soaking water
- ½ cup vegetable stock
- A teaspoon of fresh lemon juice
- 1 cup non-dairy fresh cream (preferably home-made)
- Sea salt and freshly ground pepper

Method

1) Use a wide and thick-based saucepan to heat a tablespoon of the oil over medium heat.
2) Coat the veal evenly with the mustard and season well with the salt and pepper.

3) Gently place into the hot oil and fry until browned evenly on all sides.
4) Remove from the pan and set aside until needed.
5) Put the hot water in a heatproof bowl and add the dried mushrooms.
6) Leave for 5-10 minutes to rehydrate and plump up.
7) In the meantime, heat the remaining oil in the same pan used to fry the meat and stir-fry the onions for around 6 minutes until soft and the leaves are a dull green then add butter.
8) Drain the soaked mushrooms, but retain the soaking water.
9) Add the Portobello mushrooms and the drained mushrooms to the cooking pot, increase heat to high and cook until all the liquid has evaporated.
10) Season well and add the sage, sherry, ¼ cup of the reserved soaking water, the stock, lemon juice and cream.
11) Place the veal into the pan making sure to spoon some of the sauce and mushrooms it to prevent drying out during cooking.
12) Partially place the lid on and cook for 18-23 minutes.
13) To ensure even cooking, turn the meat over once during the cooking time
14) Remove meat from the pan and cut in into 1 cm thick slices.
15) Place them back into the sauce ensuring they are fully covered with the sauce, reheat slowly until warmed through.
16) Sprinkle with the lemon infused extra virgin olive oil and serve as desired.

Tandoori Chicken

Ingredients

- 1 cup, coconut milk yogurt

- 1 garlic clove, crushed
- Peeled and grated ginger piece
- 1 tablespoon each of lemon juice and olive oil
- 1 teaspoon each of masala and ground coriander
- ½ teaspoon each of chili powder and turmeric
- 6 chicken thigh fillets, trimmed

Method

1) Mix well yogurt, ginger, garlic, lemon juice, spices, oil and salt in a large bowl.
2) Double slit the top of each thigh without cutting all the way through
3) Put chicken in mixture making sure to coat well
4) Refrigerate for 3½ hours
5) Preheat oven to 220 degrees C towards the end of the refrigeration time.
6) Place chicken in a lined dish and roast until thoroughly cooked.
7) Serve with boiled butternut.

Peppered Beef Chickoli (2 servings)

Ingredients

- 8 ounces of broccoli
- 8 ounces of peppered beef steak strips
- 2 large chicken breasts

Method

1) Spray a slow cooker with anti-stick spray.
2) Place a layer of the peppered steaks in the slow cooker, ensure they are touching but not overlapping.
3) Create a second layer using the broccoli then carefully place one chicken breast.
4) Place another layer of steak, followed by the broccoli again and then the last breast.
5) Place the last layer of steak, followed by the last broccoli layer and finally 1½ cups of water.
6) Cook on medium for six to seven hours.
7) Remove from pot and cut into pieces as desired and serve still hot for best results.

Slow Cooked Low Carb Mexi Chicken (one serving)

Ingredients

- 8 ounces chicken breasts
- 2 teaspoons seasoning
- ½ cup home-made salsa
- 1 cup grated non-dairy cheddar cheese substitute

Method
1) Butter or spray the sides and the base of the slow cooker with non-stick spray.
2) Generously season the breasts with on both sides then use spoon to put salsa on top.
3) Gently put in the slow cooker and cook on medium heat for 5 hours
4) Open pot at the end of five hours, evenly put a sprinkling of cheese on the breasts.
5) Put lid back on and cook for an additional quarter of an hour.
6) Serve as desired.

Slow Cooker Lamb Carnitas (4 servings)

Ingredients

- 2 pounds boneless lamb cut into 8 pieces
- 1¼ teaspoon salt
- 1 teaspoon chili powder and one teaspoon cumin
- 1 bay lea
- 4 thinly sliced garlic cloves
- I chopped medium sized onion

Method

1) Thoroughly combine the dry ingredients before rubbing into the meat.
2) Spray or butter a slow cooker then place the meat as a single layer into the buttered cooker.
3) Atop the meat, place the cleaned bay leaf then strew the garlic and the onions on top.
4) Cook on low to medium heat for 6 to 7 hours.
5) When cooked, place in an oven dish and bake for about 7 minutes to brown.

Zucchini Cake with Whipped Cream (serves 6)

Ingredients

- 1 small avocado
- 4 tablespoon melted clarified butter
- 4 large organic eggs
- ¾ cup coconut flour
- 4 tablespoons desiccated coconut
- 3 tablespoons crushed cranberries
- ½ teaspoon baking soda
- 1 teaspoon vanilla essence
- ½ teaspoon ground cinnamon
- 6 ounces zucchinis, grated
- 4 tablespoons whole almonds, chopped
- Non-dairy whipped cream

Method

1) Pre heat the oven to 180°C.
2) Grease a small baking tin generously or line it with a baking sheet.
3) Blend the avocado, butter, eggs, coconut flour, desiccated coconut, cranberries baking soda, vanilla essence and cinnamon in a blender until smooth.
4) Put the grated zucchinis and almonds in a large mixing bowl.
5) Remove the blended mixture from blender and add to the zucchini and almond mixture.
6) Combine thoroughly then spoon it into the prepared baking tin.
7) Bake for 22-25 minutes or until it is done. You can use the skewer test to check for doneness.

8) Remove baking tin from the oven and allow it to cool still in the tin.
9) Slice as desired and top the slices with a drop or squirt of the whipped cream and garnish to your desired taste.

Pumpkin Cake with Whipped Cream (serves 6)

Ingredients

- 1 small avocado
- 3 tablespoons melted clarified butter
- 4 large organic eggs
- ¾ cup coconut flour
- ¼ cup desiccated coconut
- 4 tablespoons crushed cranberries
- ½ teaspoon baking soda
- A teaspoon vanilla essence
- ½ teaspoon ground cinnamon
- 10 ounces pumpkin, grated
- 5 tablespoons whole walnuts, chopped
- Non-dairy whipped cream

Method

1) Pre heat the oven to 180°C.
2) Grease a small baking tin generously or line it with a baking sheet.
3) Blend the avocado, butter, eggs, coconut flour, desiccated coconut, cranberries baking soda, vanilla essence and cinnamon in a blender until smooth.
4) Put the grated pumpkin and walnuts in a large mixing bowl.
5) Remove the blended mixture from blender and add to the zucchini and almond mixture.
6) Combine thoroughly then spoon it into the prepared baking tin.
7) Bake for 22-25 minutes or until it is done. You can use the skewer test to check for doneness.

8) Remove baking tin from the oven and allow it to cool still in the tin.
9) Slice as desired and top the slices with a drop or squirt of the whipped cream and garnish to your desired taste.

Baby Spinach and Eggs (serves 2)

Ingredients

- 2 small bunches of baby spinach
- 2 large orange bell peppers
- 1 brown or sweet onion
- 4 garlic cloves, finely chopped
- 2 tablespoons olive oil
- ¼ teaspoon sea salt
- ¼ teaspoon ground black pepper
- 8 large organic eggs
- Ingredients for sauce:
- ½ cup homemade mayonnaise
- 2 tablespoons Dijon mustard
- 1 teaspoon finely chopped fresh tarragon leaves

Method

1) Prepare spinach by cutting the stem out with a sharp knife.
2) When ready, chop the leaves crosswise into ribbons.
3) Remove the top off of the peppers and cut them in quarters, top to bottom.
4) Remove the white membrane and deseed.
5) Slice the quarters again to make very thin strips.
6) Peel and cut the onion in half from top to root then slice the halves into thin half rings.
7) Heat the oil in a large stir-fry pan over medium heat, then add the onion and the peppers.
8) Fry, stirring all the time, until vegetables are soft; should take about 4 minutes.

9) Add garlic and cook for 30 seconds more, continuously stirring.
10) Season with the salt and pepper.

Savory Lentil Cake (4 servings)

Ingredients

- 3 cups brown lentils
- 1 onion, peeled
- 1 teaspoon curry paste
- 1 stock cube
- 3 tablespoons fresh coriander
- 4 tablespoons clarified butter, melted
- 1 cup coconut floor
- 4 organic eggs, boiled and sliced

Method

1) Boil lentils for 20 minutes in slightly salted water.
2) Remove from the boiling pot and place in a food processor, blend until smooth and remove from processor.
3) Place onions, coriander, pepper, melted butter, curry paste and stock cube into processor and blend until smooth
4) Remove from processor and place in a large mixing bowl.
5) Add the lentils to the processed mixture in the mixing bowl; add the flour and mix thoroughly.
6) Prepare the base of the slow cooker using a non-stick cooking paper.
7) Place half of the blended mixture in the slow cooker (the smaller the cooker the better).
8) Add the sliced eggs and place with remaining mixture on top.

9) Put the cooker lid on and cook on low heat for 3-3½ hours.
10) When cooked, remove from pot and serve with a salad of choice.

Veal and Mushrooms

Ingredients

- 1 pound veal steak, thinly sliced across the grain into ½cm thick pieces
- 1 cm long chunk fresh ginger, chopped
- 12 ounces spring greens, sliced
- 6 ounces pack sliced mushrooms
- 4 tablespoon oyster sauce
- 2 tablespoon each red wine vinegar sauce and coconut oil

Method

1) Mix sauces and set aside.
2) Heat a deep skillet until smoking hot, add 1 tsp. oil; stir-fry the meat until browned all over. Remove meat and wipe skillet
3) Add a little more oil. Stir-fry the ginger until golden,
4) Add greens and mushrooms. Stir and cook for 3
5) Add the steak and soy sauce mixture. Cook for 3 more minutes until sauce thickens a little and everything is thoroughly warmed.
6) Serve with a salad of choice

Crisp Roast Butternut

Spices help in weight loss by speeding up metabolism.

Ingredients

- 1 teaspoon vegetable oil
- 1 teaspoon ground cinnamon
- ½ teaspoon each of coriander, nutmeg
- ½ teaspoon salt
- 2lb 2 oz. butternut, cubed

Method
1) Preheat oven to 180 degrees C
2) Mix all ingredients well in a mixing bowl
3) Place mixture in oven tray and roast until soft
4) Remove from oven and serve with a salad

Slow Cooked Fish Cakes (6 servings)

Ingredients

- 1 pound hake or whiting steaks
- 2 small sweet potatoes, cooked, skinned and mashed
- 1 medium onion, grated
- 3 tablespoons chopped parsley
- 2 teaspoons lemon juice
- 2 beaten organic eggs
- 4 tablespoons coconut or hemp flour
- Sea salt and pepper

Method

1) Grease your slow cooker, one with a large base will work better
2) Place the fish into a food processor and blend slightly
3) Remove fish from processor and combine with mashed sweet potato, parsley, onions, eggs, lemon juice, flour, sea salt and pepper. Mix thoroughly
4) Place mixture on a rolling board and shape the mixture into six cakes
5) Flatten the top of the cakes slightly and put them one after the other into the slow cooker.
6) Put lid on and cook on low for five hours or so.
7) Remove from pot and place on the oven and grill for two minutes to brown.

Jicama Noodle Salad and Creamy Tahini-Ginger (serves: 2-4)

Ingredients

Dressing

- ¼ cup tahini
- 2 tablespoons toasted sesame seed oil
- Juice from a small lemon
- 1 tablespoon apple cider vinegar
- 2 minced cloves of garlic
- 1 teaspoon fresh ginger root, minced

Salad

- 2 medium size jicama roots, peeled and julienned
- 1 deseeded orange bell pepper, cut to resemble matchsticks
- 1 deseeded red bell pepper, cut to resemble matchsticks
- 1 bunch of scallions, (the white and light green parts) trimmed and cut to resemble matchsticks then sliced
- 1½ cup red cabbage, thinly sliced
- 2 cups lacinato kale, thinly sliced
- ⅓ cup cilantro leaves
- A few lime wedges
- A few hemp seeds

Method

For the dressing

1) Place the tahini, sesame oil, garlic, lime juice, turmeric, apple cider vinegar, ginger, and turmeric into a medium size mixing bowl.
2) Whisk the mixture together for 30-45 seconds then cover bowl and place in fridge until required for use.

To make the salad

1) Place the julienned jicama, bell peppers, scallions, red cabbage, cilantro, and lake into a large bowl and mix. Toss the vegetables for even distribution.
2) Share the vegetables into 2-4 large bowls.
3) Top with the dressing and enhance the color with a couple of lime wedges and hemp seeds.

Thai Chili Prawns with Courgette Noodles (2 servings)

Ingredients

- 2 tablespoon home-made fish sauce
- 1 tablespoon lime juice
- 1 large, finely minced garlic clove
- 4 tablespoons scallions, finely chopped
- 1/2 teaspoon arrowroot powder (dilute in a tablespoon cold water)
- 1 small, finely chopped, red chili
- 1 teaspoon chili powder
- 1 finely chopped shallot
- 1/2 tablespoon spirit vinegar
- 5 drops home-made Worcestershire sauce
- 13 ounces large raw prawns, deveined and butterflied
- 2 large courgette
- 2 organic eggs
- 1 tablespoon high oleic safflower oil to fry
- 2 tablespoons crushed walnuts
- 1 tablespoon finely chopped coriander
- A few lime wedges

Method

1) Create the courgette noodles using a spiralizer.
2) Put noodles on a large serving plate and set aside for later use.
3) Put the fish sauce, lime juice, garlic; vinegar and Worcestershire sauce in a small bowl and mix well.
4) Stir in the chili and arrowroot powders.
5) Use fork to break and beat egg in a small bowl.

6) Use a small wok to heat the safflower oil then add the scallions and the shallot then allow to cook as you stir continuously for the first minute of cooking.
7) Add the prepared prawns to pan and cook, stirring, until they start to turn pink.
8) Put the sauce mix in and stir for 2 minutes.
9) Force all that's in the pan to one side of the pan to leave room for the egg.
10) Pour egg onto the cleared space and cook for a minute until egg starts to set before scrambling it by mixing with everything in the pan.
11) Top the courgette noodles with the scrambled mixture and add the crushed walnuts and pepper with the chopped coriander. Garnish with lime wedges.

Grilled Salmon and Boiled Sweet Potato

Ingredients

- 1/3 cup virgin olive oil
- ¼ cup each of coarsely chopped fresh oregano and fresh lemon juice
- 4 eight ounces salmon fillets
- 2 tablespoons vegetable oil
- 1 teaspoon minced garlic
- 1 lemon cut into quarters

Method

1) Preheat barbecue to medium
2) In a small bowl, mix olive oil, lemon juice and oregano and set aside
3) Slightly rub vegetable oil and garlic into fillets and season well
4) Grill between 4-6 minutes per side
5) Serve with boiled sweet potato

Baked Sweet Potatoes

Ingredients

- 1 sweet potato (depending on the number you are cooking for)
- Olive oil to coat
- Salt and pepper to taste

Method

1) Preheat oven to 170 degrees C
2) Thoroughly wash potatoes under cold preferably running water, using a stiff brush
3) Dry potato then poke 10 to 12 deep holes using a fork; this enables moisture to escape as potato cooks
4) Place potato in a bowl and coat lightly with olive oil
5) Sprinkle all over with salt and pepper and place potato on middle oven rack
6) Bake for about an hour or until skin feels crisp and potato inside feels soft
7) Use own imagination to serve with the fruit and vegetable salad

Pesto Chicken and Brown Mushrooms on Zucchini Noodles (serves 2)

Ingredients

- 1 ½ tablespoons high oleic safflower oil
- 2 chicken breast fillets, cut into strips
- 14 ounces brown mushrooms, sliced
- 3 tablespoons basil pesto (home-made and cheese free)
- ½ teaspoon crushed garlic
- Sea salt and black pepper to taste
- 18 ounces zucchini
- fresh basil leaves to garnish

Method

1) Heat the oleic safflower oil in a stir-fry pan and stir-fry the chicken until well browned.
2) Add the mushrooms and to the pan and continue stir-frying for an additional 5 minutes.
3) Mix in the basil pesto and garlic ensuring you thoroughly combine.
4) Season well with the sea salt and black pepper and set aside until ready to use.
5) Clean the zucchini well and spiral them with a spiralizer or julienne peeper (or whatever works for you).
6) Boil two cups of salted water and blanch the zucchini spirals for two or so minutes. Drain.
7) Place the zucchini noodles on a serving plate and crown with the stir-fried chicken and mushrooms.
8) Serve with fresh basil and a salad of choice.

Rabbit Meat Panfry

Ingredients

- 14 ounces deboned rabbit meat
- 1 tablespoon coconut flour
- 2 teaspoons dried rosemary
- 3 tablespoons rapeseed oil
- 7 ounces sliced mushrooms
- 1 finely chopped garlic clove
- 1 ¼ cup vegetable stock

Method

1) Cut meat into finger-thick strips
2) Combine together rosemary, flour and some salt and pepper.
3) Dip meat into the rosemary and flour mixture and shake off any excess.
4) Heat 2 of the tablespoons of oil in a wide and thick-based frying pan and fry rabbit meat until well browned on all sides.
5) Remove from pan and set aside until ready to use.
6) Heat remainder of oil and stir-fry the mushrooms for 2 minutes or so.
7) Pepper in the garlic and place meat back into the frying pan
8) Add the stock, mixing continuously until mixture boils.
9) Simmer until meat is cooked through.
10) Serve as desired.

BBQ Chickpeas and Cilantro Humus with Asparagus, Avocado and Sweet Potato

Ingredients

For the Cilantro Hummus

- 7 ounces mixed lentils, boiled
- 2 tablespoons pecan nuts
- Juice of one lemon
- 1 minced garlic clove
- 3 tablespoons chopped fresh cilantro
- Sea salt and a good pinch of black pepper
- 1/3 cup good quality virgin olive oil

For the bowls

- 1 bunch asparagus, with ends trimmed
- 1 tablespoon virgin olive oil
- pinch of sea salt and ground pepper
- ½ teaspoon of chili powder
- ¼ teaspoon of cayenne pepper
- 1 ½ cups home-made non-corn barbeque sauce
- A medium size baked sweet potato, sliced into 1/2 inch circles
- 14 ounces boiled organic chickpeas
- 4 cups greens (personal choice)
- 1 sliced, medium sized avocado
- nutritional yeast

Method

1) Preheat oven to 200°C.

2) Make the hummus by putting the lentils, cilantro, pecan nuts, pepper, lemon juice, garlic, pepper and sea salt into a food processor.
3) Blend until smooth and scrap mixture from the sides if necessary.
4) With the blend motor running, drizzle in the olive oil until mixture becomes smooth. Add salt and pepper for taste and refrigerate until ready for use.
5) Put the sweet potato and asparagus on a baking tray and toss with a tablespoon of olive oil, sea salt and ground pepper.
6) Place tray the preheated oven and roast for 25-30 minutes, the asparagus should be tender and crisp when done, and the sweet potato should pass the fork test.
7) While asparagus and potatoes are roasting, thoroughly mix the BBQ sauce, cayenne pepper and chili powder.
8) Place the chickpeas in a medium bowl and toss with half the mixed sauces or whatever is enough to completely cover the chickpeas. Reserve any excess sauce.
9) When roasting is done, sprinkle nutrition yeast on the sweet potato and chop the asparagus in half and set both aside for later use.
10) Put the chickpea mixture into a pan and cook for between 5 and 10 minutes, BBQ sauce has to be a thick and should coat the chickpeas in a sticky way.
11) Take pan off the heat and stir in another BBQ sauce tablespoon.
12) To serve, place greens first at the bottom of the bowls then add the warm sweet potato circles, slices of avocado, asparagus and warm BBQ chickpeas.
13) Add spoons-full of the Cilantro Hummus then top with the nutritional yeast. Serve with the saved BBQ sauce.

Guacamole Burgers on Portobello Mushrooms (serves 4)

Ingredients

- 8 large Portobello mushrooms wiped clean with paper towel and stems removed
  1 tablespoon virgin olive oil
- 1 pound grass-fed and ground beef
- 1 medium size, peeled and ripe avocado
- 2 tablespoons home-made mayonnaise (check out Dr. Mark Hyman's recipe)
- 1 tablespoon lime juice
- ¼ teaspoon cumin, ground
- 1 large deseeded and diced tomato
- 1 deseeded and chopped jalapeno pepper
- 1 teaspoon sea salt
- ½ teaspoon of ground black pepper
- 1 cup of alfalfa sprouts

Method

1) Preheat oven to (200°C).
2) Place aluminum foil to line a baking sheet and set aside.
3) Glaze the top and bottom caps of the mushroom with olive oil, sprinkle a little salt and pepper before placing them gills side up first, onto the foiled baking sheet.
4) Place baking sheet in the oven, on middle level and bake for 10 minutes or so, then turn mushrooms over and bake for 10 minutes more.
5) When done, remove mushrooms, and the released juices, from the trays and place them on a plate.

6) Meanwhile, place half of the avocado in a small mixing bowl and mash with the back of a spoon or fork until smooth.
7) Add mayonnaise, cumin and lime juice and stir enable thorough mixing.
8) Cut remaining avocado into small cubes and mix it with the avocado mixture together with the diced jalapenos, tomatoes and a little salt.
9) Stir lightly to combine well then taste and add more seasoning if required. Set aside until needed.
10) Season the ground beef with remaining salt and the black pepper. Use your fingers to ensure ingredients are well mixed.
11) Quarter the beef mixture and mold into patties.
12) Heat a grill and grill the patties until they are as done as you desire then turn and grill the other side.
13) Place ¼ cup of alfalfa sprouts onto 4 of the mushroom caps, place a patty on each cap, add 3 tablespoons of guacamole and close using the remaining mushroom caps.
14) Serve.

Veal Chops with Mushrooms and Couscous

Ingredients

- 17 ounces veal chops
- 1 tablespoon hemp flour
- 2 teaspoon dried rosemary
- 3 tablespoon olive oil
- 8 ounces sliced mushrooms
- Finely chopped garlic clove
- 1 cup vegetable stock

Method

1.) Cut veal into finger thick strips
2.) Coat well with a mixture of the rosemary, flour and some salt and pepper
3.) Heat 2 tablespoons of oil in a wide frying pan and fry meat until browned on both sides
11) Remove from pan
5.) Heat remaining oil and fry mushrooms for 2 minutes
6.) Sprinkle in garlic and return meat to pan
7.) Stir in the stock until mixture boils. Simmer until meat is cooked
8.) Serve with couscous and a salad

Five Spice Salmon Fillets with Sesame Cabbage (Serves 4)

Ingredients

Salmon preparation

- 23 ounces skinned wild salmon
- ½ teaspoon crushed garlic
- ¼ teaspoon sea salt
- 1 ¼ tablespoons Chinese Five Spice
- 1 teaspoon coconut oil
- 1 tablespoon toasted sesame oil

Sesame Cabbage preparation

- A halved, cored and thinly sliced green cabbage
- 2 tablespoons macadamia nut oil
- 6 chopped scallions
- 1 tablespoon peeled and finely grated fresh ginger
- 4 finely chopped garlic cloves
- 1 tablespoon tamari
- 2 tablespoons black and white sesame seeds
- 2 tablespoons chopped fresh parsley

Method

1) Pre-heat the oven to 220°C.
2) Flip the salmon fillets so that the bloodline is upwards, trim the dark purple bloodline with a sharp thin knife if noticeable - makes the salmon taste milder.

3) Pepper the top part of the fillets with the crushed garlic, salt and a teaspoon of the Chinese Five Spice on each fillet. Set aside.
4) Heat a large fry pan over medium heat and add the macadamia nut oil.
5) When the oil is hot, add the scallions, garlic and ginger then cook about a minute, stirring all the while.
6) Reduce heat if needed so the garlic and ginger do not burn. Add the sliced cabbage to the pan. It will seem like a lot but it will cook down quickly.
7) As cabbage cooks, turn it over frequently to ensure it is well coated with the coconut oil continue stirring until the cabbage shrivels and softens.
8) When the cabbage is softened enough, stir in the tamari sauce, sprinkle with the sesame seeds and fold in the cilantro leaves.
9) Maintain the cabbage's warmth while you cook the salmon.
10) To make the salmon, heat a large cast iron skillet over medium heat for 4-5 minutes.
11) Add the oil to the pan, then add the salmon fillets, spiced side down.
12) Cook until the salmon is golden and crusted, being careful not to burn the spices, about 4-5 minutes.
13) Turn the fillets over, spiced side up, and place the pan in the oven. Finish cooking the salmon by roasting for 2-3 minutes if fillets are an inch thick.
14) Remove the pan from the oven and serve drizzle the salmon with the sesame oil and top over the cabbage.
15) For any leftovers, place in glass storage containers with tight fitting lids. Salmon is best enjoyed the next day and cabbage will keep 2-3 days

Butternut and Coconut Cake (serves 6)

Ingredients

- 5 tablespoons coconut oil
- 4 large organic eggs
- 7 ounces coconut flour
- 5 tablespoons desiccated coconut
- 3 tablespoons crushed cranberries
- An avocado
- 1 teaspoon baking soda
- 1 teaspoon vanilla essence
- 9 ounces butternut, grated
- 2 tablespoons whole walnuts, chopped
- Non-dairy whipped cream

Method

1) Pre heat the oven to 180°C.
2) Grease a small baking tin generously or line it with a baking sheet.
3) Blend the avocado, oil, eggs, coconut flour, desiccated coconut, cranberries baking soda and vanilla essence in a blender until smooth.
4) Put the grated butternut and walnuts in a large mixing bowl.
5) Remove the blended mixture from blender and add to the zucchini and almond mixture.
6) Combine thoroughly then spoon it into the prepared baking tin.
7) Bake for 22-25 minutes or until it is done. You can use the skewer test to check for doneness.

8) Remove baking tin from the oven and allow it to cool still in the tin then slice.

Sealed Hake with Olive Salsa (serves 4)

Ingredients

- 4 hake fillets
- 2 tablespoons melted margarine
- 1 cup black olives
- 1 cup thinly sliced cucumber
- ¼ cup olive oil
- 1½ tablespoon vinegar
- Salt and pepper to taste

Method

1) Heat a wide base frying pan over medium heat.
2) In the meantime, brush hake fillets with melted margarine and season well.
3) Fry the fish for 6 minutes per side or until each side is nicely browned and the inside well cooked.
4) Use a medium sized mixing bowl to thoroughly mix the olives and the cucumber, sprinkle with oil and vinegar.
5) Season well, toss and serve with a homemade sauce of choice.

Spaghetti Squash and Chickpea Sauce

Ingredients

- 1 spaghetti squash
- 2 tablespoons each of olive oil and high oleic safflower oil
- Sea salt and black pepper
- 1 small thinly sliced onion
- 4 chopped cloves of garlic
- 1 big crushed tomato
- 2 teaspoons basil, dried
- ½ teaspoon oregano, dried
- 12 ounces cooked and drained chickpeas

Method

1) Preheat oven to 190 °C.
2) Cut squash from top to bottom create two oval halves then take out the seeds and discard.
3) Rub olive oil on the flesh of the squash and pepper with black pepper and a little sea salt.
4) Place the squash cut-side-up in a baking tray and bake for 40 minutes or so, or until a fork easily goes into the flesh.
5) In the meantime, heat the high oleic safflower oil in a large thick base frying pan over medium-high heat; add the sliced onion and a pinch of the sea salt.
6) Stir here and there in the 10 minutes or so cooking time or until onion becomes clear and soft.
7) Add chopped garlic to the pan and cook for 30 seconds more before adding the tomato, oregano, dried basil and cooked chickpeas.

8) Reduce the heat to low and allow mixture to simmer gently for about 12 minutes; adjust seasoning if required then set aside until needed.
9) Take out squash from the oven and allow it to cool slightly.
10) Gently take out the flesh of the squash with a spoon; place it in a large bowl. It should look like strands of spaghetti.
11) Throw away the squash skin.
12) Serve the spaghetti squash with chickpea tomato sauce

Shawarma Chicken with Basil-Lemon Vinaigrette (serves 4)

Ingredients

Chicken Shawarma

- 1 pound free-range chicken breast
- 2 tablespoons high oleic safflower oil
- Juice from a medium sized lemon
- ¾ teaspoon sea salt
- 3 minced cloves of garlic
- 1 teaspoon of curry powder
- ¼ teaspoon of ground coriander
- ½ teaspoon ground cumin

For the Salad

- 6 cups spring greens
- 1 cup halved cherry tomatoes
- 2 handfuls roughly chopped fresh basil leaves
- 1 sliced avocado

For Basil-Lemon Vinaigrette

- 1 clove garlic, smashed
- 2 large handfuls fresh basil leaves
- ½ teaspoon sea salt
- Juice from a medium sized lemon
- 5 tablespoons virgin olive oil

Method

1) Combine olive oil, garlic, lemon juice, curry powder, cumin, sea salt and coriander then whisk briskly.
2) Cut chicken into strips 3 inches long and put in a large Ziploc bag or small sealable bag together with the whisked mixture to marinade.
3) Seal and refrigerate for a minimum of 20 minutes and if possible overnight to draw out the most flavor.
4) In due time, heat a large thick based frying pan over medium heat and add the safflower oil.
5) Add chicken to the pan and fry, turning chicken regularly, until chicken is slightly browned but well cooked and the juices are running clear, this should take about 6 to 8 minutes.
6) In a small blender, blend the salt, basil, lemon juice and garlic until smooth.
7) Add the oil gradually while the blender motor is running then blend until well combined. Set aside until ready to use.
8) For salad preparation, place the green vegies into a mixing bowl then mix with a little sea salt and ground pepper.
9) Transfer greens to serving bowl and top with the chicken along with the avocado, tomatoes and basil.
10) Drizzle the basil-lemon vinaigrette on top.
11) Serve and enjoy.

Beef and Broccoli Stir-fry (serves 1)

Ingredients

- 7 ounces sirloin steak
- 1 teaspoon cornstarch
- 2 tablespoons avocado oil
- 1 thinly sliced onion
- 3 minced garlic cloves
- 1 tablespoon minced ginger
- 4 cups chopped broccoli

For the sauce

- $^2/_3$ cup chicken stock
- ¼ cup home-made hoisin sauce
- 2 tablespoon home-made oyster sauce
- 1 tablespoon rice vinegar
- 1 teaspoon sesame oil
- 4 tablespoons cornstarch
- ½ teaspoon chili paste

Method

1) Whip all the sauce ingredients together to make the sauce. Set sauce aside until required.
2) Slice beef thinly across the grain, into strips and toss with cornstarch.
3) Heat a tablespoon of oil in deep skillet over medium to high heat.
4) Stir-fry the beef strips for 3 minutes and put in separate bowl when done.

5) Put the remaining oil into the skillet and sauté onion, ginger and garlic for 2 minutes or so.
6) Add ½ cup water and the broccoli before boiling for about 3 minutes.
7) Pour sauce in and stir continuously until the sauce thickens.
8) Add beef and any juices and cook for a further 3 minutes.
9) Remove from the heat and serve while still hot.

Caesar Salad

Ingredients

<u>Roasted Chickpea Croutons</u>

- 1 ½ cups cooked, drained and rinsed chickpeas
- 1 teaspoon of virgin olive oil
- 1/2 teaspoon sea salt
- 1/2 teaspoon dried and ground garlic
- A little cayenne pepper

<u>Caesar Dressing</u>

- 1/2 cup raw cashews
- 1/4 cup tepid water
- 2 tablespoons virgin olive oil
- Juice from a small lemon
- 1/2 tablespoon of Dijon mustard
- 1/2 teaspoon crushed garlic
- 2 teaspoons capers
- 2 garlic cloves
- 1/2 tablespoon Worcestershire sauce (home-made and gluten-free)
- 1/2 teaspoon sea salt and pepper, for seasoning

<u>For the seed and nut Parmesan</u>

- 2 tablespoons hulled hemp seeds
- 1/3 cup cashews, raw
- a garlic clove
- 1 tablespoon each of nutritional yeast and virgin olive oil

- 1/2 teaspoon dried and crushed garlic
- sea salt

For the lettuce
- 5 cups de-stemmed and chopped kale
- 10 cups chopped romaine lettuce

Method

1) Soak all cashews for 3 hours at least, but much better overnight. Drain them and rinse well.
2) Preheat oven to 200°C.
3) Place drained chickpeas in a tea towel to rub dry. Some skins might fall off but that's okay.
4) Place chickpeas into a large baking sheet and drizzle oil on them and roll them around to coat.
5) Sprinkle the garlic, salt, and cayenne then toss to coat.
6) Place in the preheated oven and roast for 18-20 minutes.
7) Roll the chickpeas gently around the baking sheet to turn them then keep roasting for a further 10 to 15 minutes. Peas should appear slightly golden when done. Set aside to cool.
8) Make the dressing by adding the cashews and all the dressing ingredients - save for the salt - into a blender and blend on high until dressing becomes extremely smooth. Add a little water if required and season to desired taste.
9) Set aside until required.
10) To make the cheese, place 2 garlic cloves and cashews into a small food processor and process until they are finely chopped.

11) Add all the other ingredients and pulse to ensure thorough combination of the mixture. Season to desired taste.
12) Place chopped lettuce into an extra-large bowl and mix with the chopped romaine.
13) To assemble, add the dressing to lettuce and romaine mixture and toss until well mixed. Season with salt then mix once more. Sprinkle the mixture onto the roasted chickpeas, and top with the Parmesan cheese.
14) Serve immediately.

Paleo Scotch Eggs

Very few snacks are as filling as Scotch eggs. You will crave very little else after eating them.

Ingredients

- 2 hard-boiled eggs
- 14 ounces sausage meat
- Garlic flakes
- 2 tablespoons coconut oil

Method

1) Mix meet and garlic
2) Thoroughly cover unshelled egg with meat mixture
3) Fry on medium heat until meat is done and browned all round

Did you know?

Eggs contain high quality proteins, folic acid and vitamin D. These increase alertness and a lack of vitamin D is associated with reduced mental function.

Snacks and Puddings

Onion Rings

Ingredients

- 1 cup home-made non-dairy sour cream
- 1 teaspoon lemon juice
- 2 teaspoon chopped green chilies
- ½ medium sized avocado
- 7 medium sized basil leaves
- Salt and pepper to season
- 1 large onion or 2 small ones
- 2 organic eggs
- 1 teaspoon of crushed garlic
- ¼ cup coconut flour
- 1 teaspoon sesame seeds
- ¼ teaspoon cayenne pepper
- pinch of salt
- 2 tablespoons olive oil

Method

1) Prepare a dip by placing the sour cream, lemon juice, green chilies, avocado, basil leaves, salt and pepper in a blender and blend until smooth.
2) Refrigerate blended mixture until ready to use.
3) Slice the onion into half cm rings.
4) Lightly whisk together the egg and garlic.
5) Soak the onion rings in the egg mixture and leave for 10 minutes.

6) Thoroughly mix the flour, cayenne, sesame seeds, and salt.
7) Heat the oil in a double base pan under medium heat.
8) Dip individual onion rings into the flour mixture, remove, shake off the excess and then place in the hot oil.
9) Fry rings in sizable batches until nicely browned.
10) Drain on paper towel and serve with the refrigerated dip.

Spicy Gizzards (serves 2)

Most spices are believed to speed up metabolism making them perfect for weight loss.

Ingredients

- 7 ounces chicken gizzards
- 1 tablespoon high oleic safflower oil
- ½ teaspoon each of ground paprika, cumin and coriander
- Sea salt

Method

1) Boil salted water, gently drop in the gizzards and cook for five minutes.
2) Remove from heat and dry the gizzards.
3) Place in a mixing bowl and mix in the spices.
4) Heat the high oleic oil in stir-frying pan over medium heat and place the gizzards.
5) Stir-fry the gizzards until they are browned all over.

Homemade Black Berry Chocolate

Spoiling yourself with chocolate once in a while makes healthy eating worthwhile.

Ingredients

- 1 cup unsweetened cocoa powder
- ¼ cup crushed black berries
- ½ cup coconut oil
- 4 tablespoons raw organic honey
- ½ teaspoon unsweetened vanilla powder

Method

1) Place coconut in a moderately heated oven in an oven proof bowl and allow to melt.
2) Remove from oven and briskly whisk in honey until it fully dissolves
3) Put back in the oven for 2 minutes, remove.
4) Add cocoa powder and whisk for two minutes, return to oven for a minute.
5) Remove from oven and whisk for three more minutes.
6) Add vanilla powder and black berries and keep on whisking.
7) Spread to desired thickness then place in fridge friendly container and refrigerate.
8) After 3-4 hours, remove from fridge and break into pieces.

Guilt-free Brussels Sprout Chips

Ingredients

- 2 cups of Brussels sprouts leaves
- 1½ tablespoons high macadamia oil
- Mixed spices
- Sea salt

Method

1) Preheat oven to 210°C
2) Combine the Brussels sprouts leaves with the oil, salt and spice; then mix well.
3) Line a baking tray with an anti-stick baking sheet and arrange leaves in single layer on the sheet.
4) Place baking tray into the oven and bake until the leaves are crispy and slightly browned in the edges
5) Serve as hot as possible.

Did you know?

Brussels sprouts significantly reduce risk of cancer, especially ovarian cancer, prostate cancer, breast cancer, colon cancer and bladder cancer.

Multi-berry Roll-Ups

Ingredients

- 4 cups chopped fresh cranberries, raspberries, wild berries and/or blackberries, pitted where necessary
- 2 teaspoons of lemon juice
- 1 teaspoon cinnamon
- 2 cups boiling water

Method

1) Place boiling water in a saucepan then add the berries.
2) Cover saucepan and boil on low heat for 10 minutes or so.
3) Remove pan lid and gently mash the berries.
4) Mix in the lemon juice and cinnamon thoroughly.
5) Boil for 10 more minutes with no lid on pan.
6) Remove from pan and place in a processor.
7) Blender until very smooth.
8) Line a baking sheet and place the blended mixture on the sheet.
9) Switch on oven to 65 degrees C, place baking sheet inside and allow the fruit mix to dry overnight.
10) Cut into good-sized pieces and enjoy.

Macadamia Nut Hummus

Ingredients

- 1½ cups chopped macadamia nuts
- 2 teaspoon garlic flakes
- 2 tablespoons lemon juice
- ½ teaspoon salt

Method

1) Place all the ingredients in food processor and blend.
2) Blend in ½ cup water and keep blending for a couple of minutes, adding water or seasoning as required or desired.
3) Remove from blender, place in a fridge container and chill for about thirty minutes before serving.

Turkey Bacon-Wrapped Eggplant

Ingredients

- Thin Turkey bacon strips
- Egg-plant, cut into chips
- 2 tablespoons high oleic safflower oil for frying

Method

1) Heat the oil in a stir-fry pan over medium heat and stir-fry the eggplant chips until well browned.
2) Remove from pan and set aside until required.
3) Use pan and remaining oil to fry the bacon strips until they are as crispy as you prefer.
4) Completely wrap the bacon strips around the eggplant chips.
5) Ensure bacon strips are intact by placing toothpicks from one side to come out on the other side, and serve.

Fried Chili Onion Rings

Ingredients

- 7 ounces almond or coconut flour
- 2½ medium sized white onions
- 2 beaten organic eggs
- 2 teaspoons each of paprika and chili powder
- 2 tablespoons high oleic safflower oil

Method

1) Slice the onions into 0.5 cm thick slices and separate into rings.
2) Thoroughly mix all the dry ingredients in a mixing bowl.
3) Dip the onion rings into the beaten egg then dip into dry ingredient mixture
4) Slightly heat the oil in a thick-based frying pan and fry rings over medium heat until golden all over.
5) Remove from heat and serve.

Sweet Potato Roast

Sweet potato snacks will keep you full for longer and therefore help you eat less and shed unnecessary weight.

Ingredients
- 2 pounds sweet potatoes
- 1 teaspoon olive oil
- Salt and pepper seasoning

Method

1) Preheat oven to 180°C
2) Wash and peel sweet potatoes
3) Slice them into chips
4) Drizzle oil and bake for 20 minutes
5) Remove from oven and season before returning to oven
6) Bake until crisp outside and soft inside.

Did you know?

Sweet potatoes are a versatile vegetable that you can enjoy boiled, fried, roasted, baked, pureed, steamed or grilled.

Nutty Butter and Berry Bites (serves 2)

Nuts are filling and will help you eat less and maintain your desired weight through helping you eat infrequently.

Ingredients

- 8 ounces dried berries chopped

- 1 cup raw nuts

- 1 cup raisins

- ½ teaspoon cinnamon

- ½ cup shredded coconut, unsweetened

Method

1) Place the nuts, raisins and cinnamon in a food processor and process for four minutes
2) Add the dried berries and pulse for 40 seconds, add the coconut and pulse for a further 15 seconds
3) Cover a cutting board with a plastic wrap and place the fruit mixture on top
4) Keeping the plastic wrap between your hands and nut mixture, press the mixture together to form one large square
5) Wrap up the square and place it in a freezer for 30 minutes
6) Cut the square into 2cm by 2cm squares using a sharp knife
7) Refrigerate in an airtight container.

Did you know?

Nuts are a great source of vitamin E that is associated with improved neurological performance and longevity.

Parsnip Chips with Truffle Oil

Ingredients

- 4 medium parsnips, peeled and sliced into chips
- 2 tablespoon each of olive oil and chopped parsley
- 2 teaspoon truffle oil
- Salt and pepper

Method
1) Preheat oven to 200 degrees C
2) Mix chips with olive oil, salt and pepper
3) Place single-layered on baking sheet and bake for 20 minutes
4) Adjust oven upwards to 220 degrees C and turn chips over
5) Bake for 8-10 more minutes
6) Place chips in bowl and toss with the truffle oil and parsley.

Did you know?

The foliate in parsnips enables them to provide vital nutrients that help fight cardiovascular disease and dementia.

Chocolate Cherry Bites

Ingredients

- 1 cup uncooked almonds
- 2/3 cup dates, dried and pitted
- 1/2 cup dried cherries
- 5-8 tablespoon cacao
- 1/4 cup uncooked pecans
- 2 pinches of sea salt

Method

1) Process the almonds in a blender until well chopped. Large pieces are okay but be sure not to blend into flour if you are to have a good texture.
2) From the processed almonds, remove about a third of a cup and set aside to use in the final step.
3) Add the dried cherries and pitted dates and process together with the other almonds. To be done, they should be finely chopped and sticky and a dough will start to emerge.
4) Add in the pecans and cacao and blend until pecans are chopped and everything well mixed.
5) Season to taste before pulsing the mixture.
6) Add in the reserved 1/3 cup slightly processed almonds and pulse together with mixture. Dough should not disintegrate, if it does, add some water, a tablespoon at a time until the dough is well formed.
7) Shape as desired and place in a fridge friendly, airtight container and refrigerate. Bites only taste good after refrigeration.

Fried Eggplant

Ingredients
- 1 large eggplant
- 3 beaten eggs
- Seasoned breadcrumbs
- Coconut oil

Method
1) Peel and thinly slice eggplant
2) Dip slices into egg then coat with breadcrumbs
3) Fry in melted coconut oil until golden brown

Did you know?

Eggplants are high in bioflavonoids, which control high blood pressure and relieve stress.

Roasted Pumpkin Seeds

Ingredients
- Pumpkin seeds
- 1 teaspoon olive oil
- 1 teaspoon curry powder
- Sea salt

Method
1) Clean and dry the seeds
2) Spread sparsely onto baking tray
3) Sprinkle oil and salt
4) Roast at 160°C for ten minutes
5) Remove from oven, stir then return to oven
6) Add curry powder in the last three minutes of cooking, ensure they do not brown

Did you know?

Pumpkin seeds are among the few foods with nutritional value e.g. protein content that improves as they decompose.

Roasted Cauliflower

Ingredients
- Small florets to equal 1 cauliflower head
- 4 tablespoons olive oil
- Salt and pepper

Method
1) Preheat oven to 200°C
2) Whisk oil and seasoning together
3) Add florets and toss thoroughly
4) Place florets on baking tray and roast for an hour, turning them at intervals

Did you know?

Cauliflower contains indole-3-carbinol, which is known to prevent prostate and breast cancers.

Vanilla and Almond Chia Pudding

Ingredients

- 2 cups home-made unsweetened almond milk
- 1/2 cupchia seeds
- 1/2 teaspoon vanilla powder
- 1-2 tablespoons raw honey
- Blackberries, raspberries and/ or cranberries
- Almonds or other nuts for topping

Method

1) Thoroughly mix together almond milk, vanilla powder and chia seeds in a mixing bowl until mixture starts to thicken.
2) Cover and store refrigerated for two to four hours but preferably overnight.
3) Check before serving, if pudding has become too thick; add a bit of water. Top with the fresh berries and nuts of choice.

Chia Tahini and Berry Pudding

Ingredients

- 1/2 cup chia seeds
- 2 cups coconut nut milk
- 1/2 teaspoon vanilla extract
- Maple syrup to taste
- 1 tablespoon tahini
- handful of fresh raspberries
- Raspberry and blackberry topping

Method

1) Thoroughly whisk together all the ingredients, preferably in a glass jar. After about 2 minutes of whisking there should be no lumps left.
2) Thereafter, allow to sit for 15 minutes then stir again.
3) Close the container and place the chia pudding in the fridge for at least 2 hours or even overnight.
4) Serve with frozen berries or your topping of choice.
5) You can create layers by making different chia seed puddings then setting them layer after layer in a jar.

Chocolate Chia Pudding

Ingredients

- 1/2 cup chia seeds
- 2 cups hemp milk
- 1/2 teaspoon vanilla extract
- Maple syrup to taste
- 2 teaspoons raw organic cacao
- 1 tablespoon coconut flakes
- A handful of chopped berries of choice
- Roasted nuts of choice (not peanuts) for topping

Method

1) Thoroughly whisk together all the ingredients, preferably in a glass jar. After about 2 minutes of whisking there should be no lumps left.
2) Thereafter, allow to sit for 15 minutes then stir again.
3) Close the container and place the chia pudding in the fridge for at least 2 hours or even overnight.
4) Serve with roasted nuts or your topping of choice.

Conclusion

I hope you have found the information in this book valuable and that the book has answered any questions you might have had about the EFGT diet plan developed by Dr. Mark Hyman.

This book explained the fat burning concept of ketosis and how this is in line with the EFGT diet and showed how the opposite is true of carbohydrate rich diets. The book additionally provides recipes for the various meals of the day to ensure you always have a proper meal in your tummy.

Good luck on your adventure to better health and wellness!

Thank You

Before you go, I'd like to say 'thank you' for purchasing my book. You could have picked from multiple books on the subject but you decided to give mine a chance.

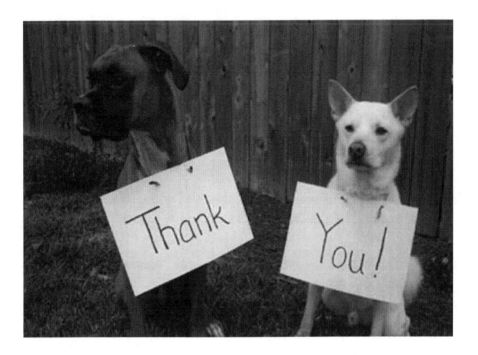

So again, thanks for purchasing my book and reading it all the way through. Now I would like to ask a small request of you, which will take about 60 seconds of your time. Could you take a minute and kindly leave a review for this book on amazon.

To do so simply go to: http://amzn.to/

This feedback will help me to continue to write books that really make a difference. So if you enjoyed it, please let me know! Thank you and good luck!

Preview Of 'Raw Food Diet - Adrenal Fatigue – Overcome Adrenal fatigue Syndrome With The Adrenal Reset Diet.' – By David Wilson'

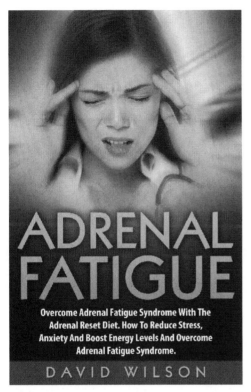

Description:

"Have you found that despite trying everything to get some much needed rest and recuperation you still have that 'wired but tired' feeling. You know the one with low-level anxiety at the same time as feeling lethargic and unmotivated? Are you finding it trickier to focus and concentrate on tasks? Are you less motivated about doing things, which you used to love? Has your sex life taken a nose-dive?

By purchasing "Adrenal Fatigue" you will be able to gain relief from the turmoil and restore your body into a state of **calmness** with a pervading sense of **ease** and **clarity** to **soothe** your mind and body. Not only that but with this **step by step** guide you will have a **clear** understanding of how the adrenal glands function when they are **fresh** and **rejuvenated**. You may not believe it now but by **letting go** and **relaxing** inside you can give your body the **deep rest** and **cleanse** that it needs. Living more **harmoniously** and in a **tranquil** state is a **solution** available to you by following this book."

Go to: http://amzn.to/1U1a1GH

David Wilson's Publications

Below you'll my other book that is popular on Amazon and Kindle as well. Simply go to the link below to find out more. Alternatively, you can visit my author page on Amazon to see other work done by me.

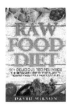 Raw Food Diet: 50+ Raw Food Recipes Inside This Raw Food Cookbook. Raw Food Diet For Beginners In This Step By Step Guide To Successfully Transitioning To A Raw Food Diet

Go to: http://amzn.to/1OgfXyJ

34521956R00094

Made in the USA
Middletown, DE
24 August 2016